Dental Patient Communication: Boosting Treatment Acceptance

DR. GERMAN GOMEZ

D.D.S., M.D., Ph.D.

DEDICATION

To my beautiful daughter and wife, who inspire me every day to become a better person and a better professional.
Their unconditional support is my biggest strength.

To my parents and brothers, whose constant faith, hope, help, and love have been a pillar for me through the peaks and valleys of my life's journe

CONTENTS

Acknowledgments   i

1   Introduction   1

COMMUNICATION BASICS   3

2   Basics of Patient Communication   3

3   What language to use for patients   12

4   The Keywords of Closing   21

5   Why asking questions is important in selling   31

6   Why the way you communicate is so important   36

THE BUYING HABITS   41

7   5 reasons patients don't buy your treatments   41

8   3 reasons why patients buy your treatments   46

PSYCHOLOGICAL RULES   49

9   The Psychology of saying Yes   49

10   Create Ideal Acceptance Conditions   58

11   Pre-suasion Principles   73

THE PROCESSES   81

12   The Closing Sequence   81

13   The 5 Steps of the Communication Process   94

	THE PRESENTATION	103
14	Basic Thoughts on Treatment Presentations	103
15	Powerful Questions during the Presentation	111
16	3 Step Technique for Patients to say Yes	119
17	Overcoming Barriers during the Presentation	123
18	Mistakes during the Case Presentation	128
	ADDITIONAL TIPS AND TRICKS	136
19	Active Listening	136
20	Gift-Wrap your Value	139
21	Small Tips and Tricks for Case Presentations	145
	THE OBJECTIONS	156
22	Your First No	156
23	A simple idea on how to handle objections	162
24	Most common Objections and how to handle them	164
	SPECIAL SITUATIONS	176
25	When the Patient asks	176
26	The Indecisive Patient	182
27	The Angry Patient	186
	ABOUT THE AUTHOR	198

ACKNOWLEDGMENTS

The contents of this work are intended to further general understanding, and discussion only and are not intended and should not be relied upon as recommending or promotinga specific method, diagnosis, or treatment by health science practitioners for any particular patient.The author makes no representations or warranties with respect to the accuracy or completeness of the contents of this work and specifically disclaim all warranties, including without limitation any implied warranties of fitness for a particular purpose. Given ongoing research, equipment modifications, changes in governmental regulations, and the constant flow of information relating to the use of medicines, equipment, and devices, the reader is urged to review and evaluate the information provided. Readers should consult with a specialist where appropriate. The fact that an organization or Website is referred to in this work as a citation and/or a potential source of further information does not mean that the author or the publisher endorses the information the organization or Website may provide or recommendations it may make. Further, readers should be aware that Internet Websites listed in this work may have changed or disappeared between when this work was written and when it is read. No warranty may be created or extended by any promotional statements for this work. The author shall not be liable for any damages arising therefrom.

Last but not least, when the author is writing about, and referring himself to the patient, the dentist or the dental team as "he", or is using the male version in an example, his intention is always to include the male, female and diverse genders.

1
INTRODUCTION

Dear reader, thank you for buying this book. It is directed to dentists or even physicians or the staff of the office, and everybody who wants to improve their communication skills.

We will talk about the communication basics, the psychological rules that are behind the acceptance of our offers, the process that we have to fulfill, the presentation techniques, tips and tricks about the presentation. Then the objections and how to handle them, and then how to handle special situations.

The moment you opened up a dental office, you started to be in business. You have all these expenses that you have to cover every month, your staff, your loans, your rents, everything.

Without a business attitude, you will not be successful. Although you might only compete against other dentists in your field and you're not in a country where real businessmen and businesswomen are involved in the dental business.

Also, if you are only competing against other dentists, it's not a bad idea to have all the skills of communication and presentation techniques, to make your patients accept your treatment offers more easily.

All this will make you successful in the future without so much effort. But usually, nowadays, we need more effort, and you have to be equipped with communication skills. And these skills are not given to you in dental school.

They are given to you with books like this. Or you have an ability by yourself and you develop these skills through time.

So, this is what we did. I am condensing all that knowledge for you in this book.

I hope you enjoy this book and you get a lot of ideas, interesting ideas, and you improve your communication skills and your treatment acceptance.

I would like to transmit information to all of you. Thank you again for reading this book, I hope you enjoy it and it provides you with some advanced knowledge and ideas.

Some chapters of this book are also part of other books that I have written. I repeat them here, as it makes sense for the overall understanding of the concepts and processes. So that this book can also stand alone as a comprehensive work by itself.

This book is not about how to present for example Veneers to the patient. The technical details are mostly known by dentists. It is about the process of the presentation. How to use the psychology, how to prepare for the presentation, what questions you should ask and how to handle objections and guide the patient to a successful close to accept the best treatment option you offer to solve his problem.

COMMUNICATION BASICS

2
BASICS OF PATIENT COMMUNICATION

In this chapter, we will talk about the basics of patient communication.

You will learn the communication patterns, tonality, and body language and what to have in mind.

You have to focus on the patient. Every time you communicate with the patient. You have to focus on him or her.

Patient communication is the basis of the whole success in your clinic. This is why there is another book, just about that. This is a sales book. And some chapters need to be in both books.

Focus on the patient. You have to break the ice. You have to solve his problems. You need to get some techniques that make you break the ice with the patient and put you in the light so that the patient perceives you as a person who wants to solve his problems.

Manage the patient flow. The greeting, the sitting in the chair, the arrangement for further follow up. All these things have to be prepared and all these things have to follow a sequence so that the patient has the perception in your office, that everything is well organized, you are well organized and your team is also.

That means the treatments are also well organized. Everybody knows what to do.

Control the patient. Since the environment ensures comfort and security he has to feel sure and secure.

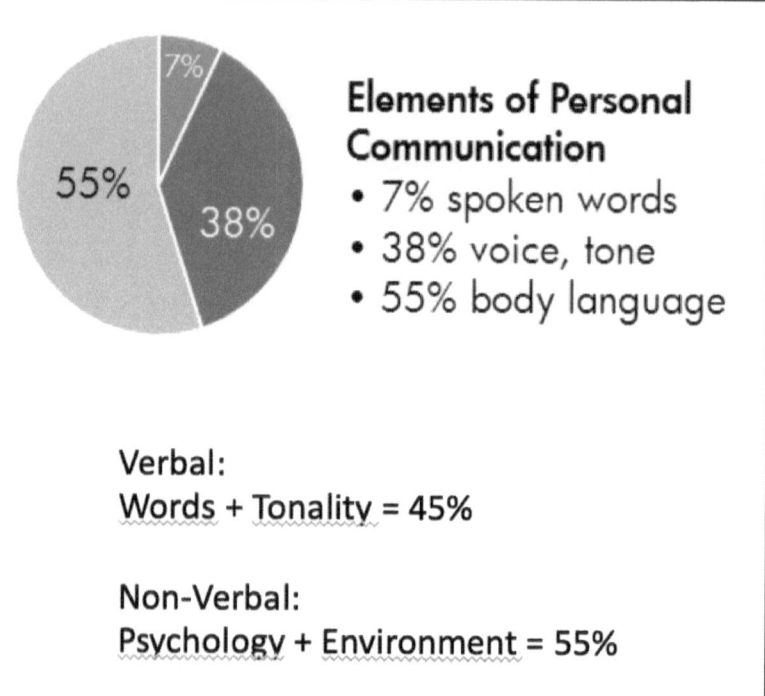

Elements of Personal Communication
- 7% spoken words
- 38% voice, tone
- 55% body language

Verbal:
Words + Tonality = 45%

Non-Verbal:
Psychology + Environment = 55%

We need to know that in communication, the spoken word is only 7% of the whole message. Inside of how you communicate with the patient is only 7% *what* you say. The rest is what you don't say. You have to control that, too.

You have to control the voice, the tone of your voice, your body language, this altogether makes 93% of the whole message.

Verbal communication is words and tonality, which is 45%.

Non-verbal is psychology and environment, your body language, which equals 55%.

You have to understand that, if we compare all the years of evolution of mankind, from Homo Sapiens or even Neanderthal to today, we have invented language just this morning, comparing

4

to the whole history with one year. Until we invented the language, people communicated with sounds, grounds, body language, and tonalities.

All these things continue nowadays also in our communication with the patient. And we have to be very conscious about it to read the patient and his body language, his tonality, his voice, and also when we have to control our body language, our voice, and our tonality.

What we say or what the patient says is only a very, very small part of what he thinks of what he communicates in reality, or what we communicate.

Let me give you an example of tonality. Tonality can change the meaning of a sentence completely depending on how I pronounce or how I give an entity to several words inside of the sentence. Here is an example sentence:

I did not say that she stole the money.

It depends on how I use the tonality, I can change the meaning. I will highlight the words, where I would give a special tone while speaking:

I did not say she stole the money.
Somebody else said it.

I did not **say** she stole the money.
I wrote it in the mail. I did not say it.

I did not say **she** stole the money.
Somebody else stole it but the money is stolen. But she didn't do it.

I did not say she **stole** the money.
I said she just took it and the money is gone.

I did not say she stole the **money**.

She did steal something, but it was not the money. She stole the toothpaste or something like that.

Do you see how it changes completely?

Also on the telephone the communication is 82% tone of the voice and only 18% the words used. Your front desk is a very important column of your office and has to be very trained in these skills.

Your vocal qualities are:

The tone. It expresses feelings or emotions.

The inflection. You emphasize words and syllables to enhance the message.

The pitch. How high or how deep your voice sounds.

The rate. How many words spoken per minute. It changes the whole thing.

The volume. How loud or soft your voice sounds.

You can play with that. And you can also hear it out when the patient talks. You have to develop listening skills in patient communication.

Let the patient make 80% of the talk and you do only 20% of the talk.

80% of the time, you need to listen and for listening, you need to develop some skills.

Do not let your mind wander when the patient is talking. Put aside personal concerns, while the patient is talking.

Do not concentrate on formulating a reply. The patient says something and you already are thinking about what to reply, and you are not focusing on what he is saying. Concentrate on what the patient is actually saying. Later, you think about what to reply, you can make a pause. You say, "let me think about it one second", and then you think about it. There's nothing bad about it. You don't have to, in a rush, answer immediately to the patient.

That seems aggressive even.

And look, as well as you listen. Don't look down. While you listen to the patient really look at him. Pick up both, the verbal and the nonverbal information that the patient is transmitting or sending to you.

Select the words that will not frighten, intimidate, or upset a patient. What words to use is another chapter, but it's important to know that you have to select words to avoid negative effects.

It sounds very logical but a lot of people do that.

Nonverbal communication is body language. The messages we send, the messages the patient senses. With our body language, the way we carry ourselves and move, our gestures, tone of our voice, facial expressions.

We can express without saying it: "I don't believe you". "Oh, that is very interesting". "Oh, that is very serious and sad".

You need to train these facial expressions. I know we are not movie stars. But we need to train our communication with the patient and show to him that we care about him. And if you train that well enough, you can transmit it not only in words, that you care but you also show that you care.

That is perceived much more than if you say it. If you only say it but you don't show it, it's like you said it without meaning it and no patient will buy from you, because no patient buys from you that you care.

In nonverbal communication, we can distinguish low-level communication from a high-level behavior.

These are different messages we want to communicate to the patient and the way how not to do it (low-level behavior) and the way how to do it (high-level behavior).

Empathy.

If we want to communicate empathy, frowning, resulting from a lack of understanding is not a good idea. If you do that, then

7

you don't show empathy.

Positive headnotes Saying "Yes". Facial expressions that reflect the content of the conversation if the conversation is sad, you cannot laugh, if the conversation is happy, then you smile and you go with the rhythm of the patient.

If Respect and warmth is your message.

Low-Level behavior would be mumbling, a patronizing tone of voice, apathy, fidgeting signs indicating the desire to leave, like looking at your watch while the patient is talking.

I know this all sounds very logical, but a lot of dentists don't have that in mind. You have to be aware of it. You know that, but you have to become aware of it.

High-level behavior would be devoting full attention, smiling, if the conversation is not sad and physical contact, show empathy, show respect, show warmth.

Genuineness.

If you avoid eye contact the whole time, the patient might think: "What's wrong with this guy? He doesn't look me in the eye. He doesn't look me in the face, what is he hiding?".

High -level behavior would be congruence between verbal and nonverbal behavior. If you say, "I feel you", you should transmit with your whole body, with your whole expression, with the whole tonality exactly that.

Confrontation.

Low-level behavior, pointing a finger or shaking a fist. Speaking with a loud tone of voice.

High-level behavior, speaking in a natural tone of voice. If you disagree with the patient, you just tell that with a natural voice. "I disagree in that point" not only "I disagree".

While there are a multitude of patient needs, there are six basic needs that stand out. We need to know these needs to cater to them so that our communication will be more effective, the patient will feel much better with us, and then at the end, we can sell much better.

Basic needs of the patient:

1 Friendliness
Basic courtesy and politeness, being warm and caring.

2 Empathy.
The patient needs to know that the dentist appreciates his wants and circumstances and provides personal attention. You need to show empathy. And the patient needs to perceive it.

3 Efficiency and punctuality.
The patients want to feel they are respected. If you let the patient wait hours and hours or even only half an hour or 20 minutes in your waiting room, that is disrespectful. I know that schedules cannot be precisely foreseen and managed, but you really need to try to plan a lot of time for every patient. I know this is not very cost-effective, but then you have to raise your prices. It's very important that you have enough time and the patient comes in punctual in your office.

We pride ourselves on not letting any patient wait in the waiting room. They are seated at their time of appointment, virtually every time.

4 Control.
The patients want to feel that they are an important part of their own treatment plan. What do you have to say is, "I will explain to you all the options so that you can make an educated decision on what to do. I can advise you, I'm your advisor and I'm the executor. I'm not the decision-maker, you make the decision." or "we together can make the decision". So he is an important part of the treatment plan. He feels he is a part of it.

5 Options and alternatives.

The patient wants to know what treatment options are available. Explaining the options thoroughly is very important. I've learned in dental school that we have to explain always three options. If we don´t find three options, there is always one alternative: not doing anything. At least this option is always possible, but what happens then?

You have to explain to the patient if you don't do anything this and this may happen. But usually, you can offer three different options to solve the problem. If you only come up with two, then the third would be not doing anything.

Here is an example of three different options in Bleaching:

	Type	Product	Method	Procedure includes	Price
In- Office		with lamp	one session in the office about 1 hour	-Plaque removal -Fläsh procedure 32% -Trays -Post-treatment	X €
Combined		combined lamp and take-home	1 hour in-office + 1 week at home	-Plaque removal -Fläsh procedure 6% -Trays -Post-treatment -Take-home gel	X €
Take-Home		individual tray	2 weeks at home	-Plaque removal -Trays -Take-home gel	X €

6 Information.

A basic need of the patient is information. The patient wants to know about fees and services but in a pertinent and time-sensitive manner. Of course, he needs to know how much it is, and how long it will take and how many times he will be in our office.

Meeting the patient's needs:

You need to have a positive atmosphere, you need to show sincerity. Be sincere, show respect. I cannot stress it out enough times, patients don't like to wait. If you make a patient wait, you destroy a lot of your professionalism and of the patient's perception of you as a professional and of the clinic or the office as a professional institution. Show respect.

Respect the patient's time, resolve complaints and misunderstandings, remain approachable. Respect the patient's confidentiality. If you do that, you meet the patient's need, and this is the basis of all communication, the basis of the whole sale.

To finish this chapter, here is the image of the ideal dentist from the patient's perspective. How should the ideal dentist be:

Confident. The dentist's confidence gives me (the patient) confidence.

Empathetic. The dentist tries to understand what I'm feeling and experiencing and communicates that understanding to me.

Humane. The dentist is caring, compassionate, and kind.

Personal. The dentist is interested in me, interacts with me, and remembers me as an individual. I'm not a number. I'm not the filling in the front guy.

Frank. The dentist tells me what I need to know in plain language and a forthright manner. No technical words, no difficult things that nobody understands, except if you have gone to dental school.

Respectful. The dentist takes my input seriously and works with me. With input I mean my objections. If I have an objection, the dentist is open to my concerns.

Thorough. The dentist is conscientious and persistent.

3
WHAT LANGUAGE TO USE FOR PATIENTS

In this chapter, we want to talk about what language to use for your patients. You will learn how to replace negative words with positive words, and what are the mistakes in communication.

Words make a big difference. You have to start transforming your vocabulary. Instead of using certain words that produce a barrier, that produce the trigger, something negative in the patient's mind.

You need to start using words that are either indifferent or positive.

Here are some examples. Transform:

but *into* and

There is a difference between saying: "You are right, *but* I think ..." and saying "You are right, **and** I think ..." And this applies to all the examples. So, transform:

however *into* **and**,

try *into* **will**,

should *into* **must**,

I was wondering if *into* **I recommend** that...,

I failed *into* I am **learning**,

you might want to consider *into* I **highly recommend,**
I may be able *into* I **will,**
Do you have any questions? *into* **What question do you have?**

Here is a list of words that you should use if you feel that your patient is afraid, learn them by heart, and apply them. These are words and sentences that are made by psychologists. And they work.

For **afraid patients** use
How do you feel?
We take our time. (you calm down everything with this, you pace down everything).
I promise you.
Can I help you?
What do you fear?
Tell me honestly, what you fear.
We take good care of you. They must be sure. They must be certain. Remember, they buy certainty in an uncertain world.

For **arrogant patients:**
patients who know it all are very arrogant. They need to hear several things and then you are their best friend. Although you want to tell them "you are wrong". Don't say that directly. Use other words to do that.
"We appreciate your opinion a lot." This helps them to feel important. Arrogant patients want to feel important. That is their problem. That is why they are arrogant. Other words:
"Can we do something special for you?" Special! They need to feel special.
"You certainly know about the subject", praise the arrogant patient.
"I have special information", and then show him why he is wrong without saying it directly to him. So, you praise him and then you give him some extra information, special information.

And with that, you tell him, that, what you say is your opinion on the subject.

"We find out where our error was." You don't say "we made an error" The arrogant patient is complaining. You need to buy time.

"This is certainly very important". Remember they want to feel important.

"Your opinion or your critics is/are very important for us".

"You are very important to us."

"We try the best for you." They want to feel special, they want to feel great. They want to feel good over everybody.

"What do you think about this?" Let him give you his opinion. They want to speak, they want to decide they want to be the middle-point of everything.

"I share your opinion"

"Your treatment is very important" because he's a very important person.

Depressed patients.

Depressed patients need to hear or listen other words, for example.

"This has been proven a lot". They look for certainty.

"This will work well for sure"

"See it this way", take it to a positive site

"We help you with this"

"We understand that you are concerned"

"Take your time"

"We could solve it for example like this way.."

"We have made very good experiences with this." They look for certainty.

"You are lucky today". This raises their mood.

"Today is going especially well"

"Today it looks especially good".

Everything you say here helps a depressed patient again. Learn these sentences by heart, know with which patient you can use them, and then use them.

Aggressive patients.

You are obviously very angry.

This has made you for sure very angry (show empathy, show that you, although you disagree with why he is angry, you need to show that you understand that he's angry. You know he is angry, you confirm he is angry, and then you state, that you want to look for a solution).

I can imagine how angry you are.

Can we speak calmly about it?

I will check exactly where the error has been.

Can you describe exactly what makes you so angry?

Probably, I would be angry too in this situation.

Good that you have told that.

We take your disappointment very seriously.

Please tell me what makes you so angry. (Then they can explain.)

All these things are important for communication and selling. This chapter is in both books.

Try to avoid negative words in your conversations. Change them, and use positive or neutral words.

Sell - to **get**, to **own**, or to become.

Sign - **confirm**, **accept** (instead of sign here, say accept here, please. Or please confirm here.)

Cost or you pay - you **invest**. (it suggests, that this is a wise decision. It's a long-term thing, it's good.)

Negative expressions like:

This is not true.

You are wrong.

That is not correct.

I know that better.

I have to correct you here.

I cannot agree with you.

Don't use them, change them. Positive expressions for this would be:

- Seeing it your way, you are surely right. (and then you can go on with according to my information… and then you state your standpoint).
- Interesting opinion ….according to my information or according to my knowledge….
- Seeing it this way. It is correct…. and according to my knowledge, and then you say the opposite.
- I understand… and according to my knowledge,
- I haven't seen it this way, my opinion on that is … and then you explain how you would proceed.
- According to my many years of experience, I would do this and this or I recommend to do this and this.

These are positive expressions to act or to talk against a patient that has told you the wrong things.

Errors in communication. Don't use these sentences:
- You have to do this.
- You have to do it this way. Use instead of that: you **could maybe** do it this way, or **we try together** to do it this way.
- You should take care of… say here: it would be good to be a **bit more careful**.
- I have to do this and this on you. Say: **a solution** would be to do this and this on you.
- That is wrong. Instead of that, say: if you would do it like this, it **would be better** …
- This does not look good. For example: oh, this tooth does not look good. Don't put the patient in a state of being afraid or uncomfortable. Instead of that, use a mirror or use something to show him and say: did you **notice** this here? That is a completely different thing.
- You don't brush your teeth at all? Don't say that. Say: here you have some areas that **could be improved**.

Here are some effective words for patient interaction:

- Instead of: pain, say discomfort. Instead of: this treatment will be painful, you say that this treatment can include a little bit of **discomfort.**
- Instead of shot, say anesthetic. In the beginning, I will give you some anesthetics or **numbing liquid.** Then the patient doesn't see the needle in his mind. If you say shot he sees the needle.
- Say **remove** instead of pulling out.
- Instead of drill, say: **prepare the tooth.**
- Instead of filling, say **restoration.**
- Instead of false teeth, say **denture.** Patients understand that much better and they don't have the feeling of these fake or false teeth that don't look good. You hear false teeth and it already doesn't look good.
- Instead of operatory you say **treatment area.**
- Instead of waiting room you say **reception area.** Remember? Nobody has to wait.
- Instead of x rays say **radiographs.**
- Instead of prep and seat, a complete **two-step procedure.**
- Instead of composite or inlay say **tooth-colored restoration.**
- Instead of policy, you say **guidelines.** Policy is too strict, guidelines is something smoother.
- Instead of work, say **treatment.**
- Instead of pay, say **take care of** or **invest.**
- Instead of recall, say **continuing care.**
- Instead of buy, say **own, invest,** take it home with you take advantage of this, **move forward.**
- Instead of, well, do you want to buy it? You say, do you want to move forward with it, with the treatment?
- Instead of do you want to buy the treatment? You say, do you want to invest in your smile?
- Instead of contract, (they think they sign their life away if

they hear the word contract), you say **agreement**, (the patient thinks, ok, we can agree on something).
- Instead of contract you can say also **paperwork**, let's get the paperwork out of the way. Agreement or paperwork.

Never say: we are better than the competition, don't ever put down the competitor. Even if it is a fact. They (patients) should come to their own conclusion that it is true. Don't talk bad about the competition. Although you see, they made a really bad work in the mouth. That is what I learned in dental school. Please consider they are our colleagues. And being our colleagues, they have learned the same things. We have learned the same profession. They know what is correct.

There is a reason why this work is not correct now. You don't know how it was before. You don't know under what conditions your colleague had to make that work. And you don't know how it looked immediately after he made that work.

So, we cannot judge the work of a colleague in the mouth we can only judge how it is now, and what is the situation of the mouth now. Including the work of the competitor, yes. But how it is now, that does not necessarily mean it was badly done. Do not talk badly about others, although you might be 100% sure it was because of a bad technique or because of bad material.

Avoid technical words.

You may need to have those thirds removed. Thirds? What patient knows what thirds are? Instead say: your **wisdom teeth** need to be removed.

Tartar. Nobody knows what that is. There's a very heavy buildup of calculus on your teeth. Who knows what calculus is? They think it's calculating something. There is a very heavy buildup of **stone** on your teeth.

Tooth number 30 will be will need endo or tooth number 3.6 will need endo or tooth number 1.6 will need endo. Instead of that, say that the **second from the back on the lower right** will need root canal treatment.

Instead of quadrants say: in dentistry, we divide your mouth into four **corners.**

Instead of deep scaling or periodontal scaling say: **gum therapy**, that includes numbing the gums and cleaning out bacteria that have built up on the roots of the teeth.

Instead of anesthetic say **numbing medication.**
Instead of topical anesthetics, a **numbing gel**, or numbing rinse.

Instead of bonded filling and composite filling, say **white filling.**

Instead of explaining a product by its name say **what it does.** Example: I'm going to apply Gluma™ to this sensitive area, say, I'm going to apply a liquid desensitizer to this area.

You may feel this is an oversimplification of what we do, but it gives patients a place to start their understanding process.
We can always add details as the patient understanding increases.

Persuasion words.
Persuasion words work in the subconscious mind of the patient.
You say **introducing** instead of offer. You say, let me introduce you to this new treatment we have here. In the subconscious mind, it triggers a positive emotion.

Investment instead of paying. They invest in themselves.

Yes. Use this word now and then. 'Yes' is a good persuasion word. Every time we use yes, it triggers a positive emotion if the whole time.

Step by step. It sounds easier, not complicated. Let's make it step by step.

Now. Now creates a sense of urgency. If you use now several times in the presentation, then it creates in the patient a sense of urgency without being pushy.

You use it as much as possible: say a lot of times is the **name of the patient** or **you**.

4
THE KEYWORDS OF CLOSING

In this chapter, we will talk about the keywords of closing. You will learn the trigger words, the looping words, and the closing words.

The keywords of closing can be divided into three groups.
- trigger words,
- looping words and
- closing words, which is more the tonality that we use. That is more important than the words we actually use in closing.

<u>Trigger words</u> are short, simple words that have the ability to influence, persuade, and motivate people. We use them to get our patients to make the buying decision.

<u>Looping words</u>, involve going backward to resell the patient on you, the treatment, or the team. If there is an objection and you need to go backward in the process. In order to make this transition back to the presentation, you use certain words. These are looping words that give you the possibility to loop back. They move the patient closer to the sale.

<u>Closing words</u> which are more the tonality. The nearer you get to the close, the more important it becomes to use the right tonality. This is something that is psychologically proven.

I will just tell you the keywords that are psychologically proven for closing.

Trigger words

Trigger words, words that cause patients to react in a certain way. They are small and unnoticed by the patient. They trigger things inside of their minds and subconscious, so that they consciously make a decision.

<u>Virtually</u>

For example, we can use the word virtually. Virtually is a hedge word. It allows you to make a bold claim without speaking in absolutes. It protects you also from a legal standpoint.

Let me give you an example. Making a bold claim: My patients never have problems.

Well, first of all, the patient wouldn't believe you. And second of all, it's probably not true. So, instead of saying my patients never have problems, you can say my patients *virtually* never have problems.

You say the same thing. But "virtually" makes it much more believable and legally defensible. You didn't say they never have problems. You said, they virtually never have problems. Do you know what I mean?

So virtually is a word that you can put in to make bold claims without talking in absolutes, but you transmit the information in a form that it looks like it would be absolutely a fact. So, use virtually to avoid speaking in absolutes.

Very few things happen always. A lot of things happen virtually always.

Only

Another trigger word is only. It is a minimizing word. It is a minimizer especially when associated with price, time, number of sessions, or appointments. When you ask for treatment acceptance and include a money amount, use "only". Always!

It's only 500 Euros
sounds a lot more reasonable than
it costs 500 Euros.

It minimizes the impact of the price, the impact of time, the impact of sessions. For example, we can do all this in only two weeks or only three months, or only three sessions.

It is much better to say that than to say we can do all this in three months. If you say it with "only", then it sounds much better for the patient.

Because

"Because" is a justifying word. It provides a reason that causes people to think differently about what you are asking for.

Let me give you an example. There has been a psychological investigation with a lot of people a lot of times in different spots making the same thing, I think it was a very busy copy machine where there was always a line in the university.

And somebody comes to the line and says to the first one in line "Can I cut in the line?" in only 25% of the cases he was allowed to cut in. Just because he asked for cutting in.

If he says "Can I cut in the line because I'm in a rush", all of a sudden 75% let this person get in, only because he was in a rush, there was a reason for it.

Another time, many times they changed the cause. "because I need to" doesn't make any sense, but it was reason enough for 75% again (!) of the people to let this person cut in the line.

So, it is not important what the "because" is. It's only important that you have a reason, and you show a reason, and you use "because" to justify that reason.

It changes completely the mind of the person who receives the message. Use it when you need to justify what you are asking for and why you need it when you are closing.

Investment

Another trigger word is "investment". It is a reframing word.
It gets the patient to look at the cost of the treatment in a different way.

Your treatment doesn't cost anything. It is an investment. So, you don't use "cost". You use investment instead of cost.

It costs 500 Euros. No!
It is an investment of 500 Euros.

Use investment instead of cost.

I would be glad to

Another trigger word is "I would be glad to". It is also a reframing word.
It is powerful for the moment after a patient asks a question, and you don't know the answer.
Instead of saying "I don't know, I have to look it up". This would destroy your image of an expert. The one who knows everything in and out, this picture is what you need in his mind.

You have to use other words. To really close smoothly, don't say that. Instead, use

"I'm not sure about that. I would be glad to research it for you".

There is a difference between "I don't know" and "I'm not sure". You suggest, that you know it, but you are just not completely sure.

This, again, changes the game completely. It is a huge rapport builder, it is the positive sentence in a negative situation. You will do something for him, you research something for the patient.

Looping words

When you start getting near the close, but you see the patient isn't quite ready, you have to go back to your presentation because he came up with an objection or with a concern.

And to do that, you use different words.

Does it make sense to you?

To find out a little bit more about the concern. Your tonality should be in a calm and curious tone.

Does the idea make sense to you? Or
Do you like the idea?

True beauty

Another word is "the true beauty".

You see the true beauty of the smile design is that it fits perfectly your face, lips, and overall look.

The true beauty of the treatment is that ….

You can also use the pain points you found while asking questions. Imagine he doesn't like one of his teeth.

Then you cater to that by saying: the true beauty of this treatment is that it fixes small teeth perfectly or in a perfect way.

The patient will think: "Oh, that is exactly what I need."

The true beauty is…and then you state, how the treatment solves these problems. The problems that you found out when you asked.

As far as to my team

As far as to my team is another looping word or sentence. It is a useful transition from selling you to selling your team.

I pride myself on doing this and that and as far as to my team, I'm proud that they are doing this and this and that.

As far as to my team… and then use positive things like
- their training,
- the customer service they deliver,
- the enthusiasm they have,
- the empathy they show with the patient,
- the passion,
- the excellence they perform.

The patient has to be sold on you, on the treatment, and the team. If he has been sold on all these things, then the close is easy.

We can start off small

Another looping word, we can start off small. This is a pattern for minimizing the patient's fears but does not mean lowering the price.

You still keep the price you just start off small. In the mind of the patient there is less risk for him.

We start with a bleaching, see how it works out, and then we move on to the veneers.

Please don't take my enthusiasm for pressure

Another looping word or sentence is "please don't take my enthusiasm for pressure".

If you feel that the patient is feeling pressured, he respects if you say don't take my enthusiasm for pressure.

Now all of a sudden, this negative feeling that he has, because he feels pressured by you to make a decision turns around and he is more relaxed, he respects that.

Otherwise he still may feel pushed. Use this sentence if you see, that the patient is feeling pressured.

I see/hear/feel what you are saying

Another looping sentence is "I see/I hear/I feel what you are saying".

Don't say "I understand", because if it is an objection, you want to give the patient the impression, that you understand without actually saying that you understand. Because in reality, you don't understand why he will not buy, you know what I mean? Remember? You are absolutely convinced, that it would be the best thing on Earth, that could happen to the patient. So, you are supposed not to understand why he is giving that objection.

But you can feel, you can hear, you can see what he's saying.

You show caring and empathy. And then you loop back to the presentation, and you start reselling you, your team and your treatment, or one of the three, when you feel that the objection is aiming at one of the three things, either you, your team or the treatment.

Closing Words

Closing words, choose the ones or variations that go with your style. You have to be comfortable.

Believe me-style.

Personally, I don't believe a lot in the Believe me-style. But

Believe me,
or trust me,
if your smile gets half as beautiful as the rest of our patients, you are going to be very, very impressed.

This is one way. I don't think people will trust somebody only because this somebody says "trust me".

Obviously, psychologically, it's a keyword. And there are a lot of people or a lot of dentists who are using this style, and they have good results with that. And then you continue:

All I ask is after your smile is beautiful, I want a ton of referrals. Sounds fair enough?

Here what you are doing is you tell the patient to trust you, it's going to be really great, and because you are so sure that it is going to be so great, you want referrals from him.

So, you are sure it's going to be great this gives certainty to this patient. And in return, you want referrals from that patient, a lot of referrals and you ask if that is a fair enough.

Now you do not concentrate the patient on the closing of the treatment. You concentrate the patient on if that is fair, if he refers a patient to you, after you have made the smile beautiful.

In reality, you have overcome the step of deciding whether or not he does the treatment.

Getting started is very simple

Another losing word or sentence is "getting started is very simple". It's an excellent soft or trial close. It suggests to the patient that he's not really making the whole treatment, we're just starting and that is simple.

In reality if you start, you are going to do the whole treatment, but the suggestion to the patient is that it only is a trial. It feels only like a trial, but in reality, it is the close of the whole treatment.

Getting started is very simple. We just make now some pictures of your smile and an impression of your jaws. And we are already set.

Very simple. Let's do A, B, and then C.

Your wife/husband

Your wife or husband closing words.

Your wife or husband will be kissing you when you walk through the door.

Your wife or husband will be delighted when he or she sees your smile.

It works on the fear, that loved ones will disapprove the buying decision. Most of the patients are afraid to do a bad decision. And they are more afraid of what their partner will say, or any loved one of the family.

Here you work on this fear they have deep inside of them. And you give them the certainty of a good outcome.

Variation of Believe me-style

A variation of the Believe me style is I'm not getting rich here. You insinuate a small margin, but a long-term relationship and getting referrals. You start:

I'm not getting rich here,
but I know your smile will look really good.
And you will give me a ton of referrals
and that is how my business grows.
Sounds fair enough?

The end is like the "believe me style" and it works on certainty. You are so certain that it will be really good that you will ask him for referrals later. And this gives him also certainty about the outcome.

5

WHY ASKING QUESTIONS IS
IMPORTANT IN SELLING

In this chapter, we will talk about why asking questions is important in selling you will get to know why we have to make some questions, what is the aim of these questions and what we have to find out.

Asking questions is part of a whole own book about patient communication. This book is about selling, and you should ask questions as much as you can when you are selling.

Questions hook the mind of the patient. You are in control of a conversation if you ask questions. You can direct his mind into a certain direction with the questions you make.

Questions help also to discover the needs of the patient. They help to gather information you could use later in the sales conversation, when you want to show the value of your treatment. The value of the treatment is higher for the patient, if it meets exactly his or her needs. For you to show that the treatment caters or meets the needs of the patient, you have to find them out. You need to ask the patient to explain to you his needs.

You have to ask questions. What questions to ask and how to ask? That is another story, a whole other book. But at least I will give you some sample questions here in this book so that you can at least do something in gathering information. It's not difficult.

You need to understand, we need these questions to see what the needs of the patients are. And we use this information later when we want to present our solution. It helps us to show that this solution is exactly for him or her. This raises the value of your solution a lot, because, if it is useless for him, the value is zero.

Don't mix up value with cost. The cost is a price that you put on the treatment, the value for a patient might be higher than the cost or lower than the cost. If it is lower than the cost, he will not buy it. If the value for the patient is higher than the cost, he will buy.
You need to raise the value of your treatment in the eyes of the patient. For that, you need the information of what he needs.

One of the sales mistakes is that you talk too much in the presentation. You need to reduce your talk. I repeat this over and over again. You should do 20% of the talking and 80% should do the patient. You should listen 80% of the time.
You talk too much about the features and benefits of the treatment but what you really should do, is to find out what the patient needs, what his pain points are. You don't sell with your mouth by talking. You sell with your ears by listening. That is a ground rule of selling.

Concentrate on what you know about your patient. And if you don't know anything, find out as much as you can. How? With questions.

Find out:
His needs.

His pain points.

Not real pain. It is more: What does he want to get rid of? The motivation is much higher to run away from bad things than to run towards good things. A patient is more likely to make veneers because he has really bad looking teeth versus because he wants a beautiful smile.

Do you understand the difference? In this case his pain point is: I have really ugly teeth. And this motivates much more to do something about it, than the fact, that he can get a beautiful smile. This is something they don't really appreciate so much. They appreciate much more to get rid of their pain points.

His Why.

Why does he do something? Why does he want to do something about it? Maybe he wants to change his smile. And you think it's because of his large canines. And it's not. Just because *you* think it, it's not necessarily the real reason. That doesn't make it true.

You have to listen and understand why the patient wants to change the smile. Maybe he loves exactly these long canines. And he wants to keep them. In the new smile, they should be included.

But let us suppose he wants to change something else that maybe for you does not seem so important, but for him, it's the most important thing in the world.

You need to take that pain point and you cater to this pain point with your solution. You say these veneers will make this and this (the pain points of this patient) disappear and we will keep your long canines.

To be able to explain this, you have to find out his needs, his pain points, and his why.

Why does he want to do something about it? Maybe it's not the same thing that you think at that moment.

And of course, you have to find out if he's able and **qualified**

to pay. If he cannot pay, it doesn't make sense to do the treatment. If he cannot pay immediately, you need to look for financial solutions. Like a down payment, and then a monthly payment or something like that. Or third party financial solutions.

And find out if he has any kind of **urgency**.

All these things have to be found out with the questions. And you have to listen and use paper and pen and write it down.

You do that, because you want to use exactly these words later when you present your solution. You want to **mirror** the exact words the patient used when you are going to close.

If he hears the same words he used, he feels deeply understood. You understood him completely. You! Not any other dentist, you! You are the first one who really understood why he's doing that.

And you are the one that will give him the correct solution. That is the feeling of the patient. Use the same words. Exactly. That is why you want to use paper and pen to write down what he says.

By the way, this also shows to the patient, that you are listening and that you are concentrated in himself. There is no way that you write down something and think about something else. Our brain is not programmed for that. That means you really are concentrating on the patient's words.

Is it better to use a pen and paper or instead of that a computer? Typing is irritating for most patients, so write it down, pen and paper, pencil and paper, but write it down. And then use it later in your presentation and your close. Use his words to show that your treatment is the correct and the best for this patient. Because it caters exactly to the words he said.

If you don't know how to ask or how to continue the questions it might help you to know, that new questions come from what the patient is telling you.

He tells you something and then you continue from there. You just say:

Tell me more about that.

If you didn't understand what he meant, if you think there is something else behind what he just said, you say:

Tell me more about that.
Oh, interesting. Tell me more about that.
I see. Tell me more about that. And so on.

If you don't know what to ask, that is a good question to keep the patient talking and telling you all you need to know.

Remember, you have to find out all the needs, the pain points, his why, if there is urgency, if he can pay, and so on.

6
WHY THE WAY YOU COMMUNICATE
IS SO IMPORTANT

In this chapter, will talk about why the way you communicate is so important for your office.

You will learn what figures and data you have to trace and screen in the office. And you will learn the difference for the office between average and good communication skills.

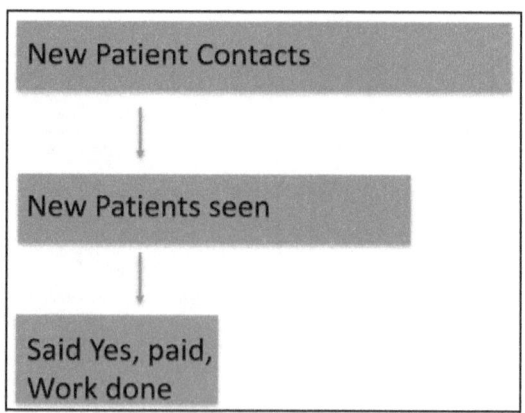

What you see in the image is the sales funnel of your office. And this is exactly what you have to trace and screen.

That means you have to know exactly the numbers. You have to know the number of new patients calling or contacting the office in different ways. Such as per email, website-chats, WhatsApp, through your Social Media or just walking in to the office and asking a question. Patients that contact your office because of word of mouth or because of your advertisement, your marketing, your online or offline marketing.

People that contact your office for information, then, apart from this number, you need to know how many of these people you have actually seen in your office.

That means how many of these new patient contacts are converted into new patients seen in your office.

And this depends completely on the communication skills of your front office, telephone skills, communication skills. I want you to understand that this is also extremely important that you make that happen and train them to be very efficient in converting contacts into actual appointments.

Then, from these new patients that you see, how many of these new patients really make the treatment with you?

These are patients that say yes to your treatment options, that have paid, and the work is done. What is the number?

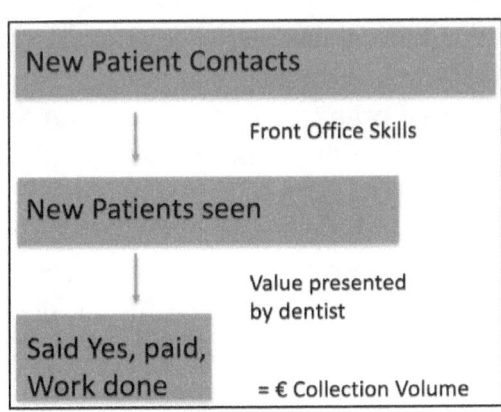

In the sales funnel, you measure how many you convert in

every step. You need to know all these figures. If you have these data you know what and where you can improve something.

This last step depends completely on your communication skills. The communication skills of the dentist or the hygienist. Let me give you an example: if from the new patient contacts, which is 100% of the figure, you have 100 people contacting.

Let us assume, that the front office converts from these 100 people that contact you for information 70%. The front office can usually not convert 100% of these people, because some people call and ask for prices and these prices are higher than other dental offices and so they go to the other dental offices. They are shoppers. Imagine the front office converts 70%.

And out of this 70%, which is not a bad number for a dental office, out of the 70%, the dentist converts 70% into accepting patients. Into patients that pay and the work has been done.

Then let me explain to you a little bit about the situation. Imagine new patient contacts are 100 people that contact. Like this the calculation is very easy.

Imagine the average amount spent by a new patient in your office is 1000 euro. This is just for you to understand the calculation and the numbers that come out. With these numbers 100,000 or 1000 is not important right now. But important is to see the difference of numbers that come out at the end for you if you compare two different communication skills or levels of skill.

Imagine that these 100 people call in a period of time, a period of one month, two months, three months, it depends on the office, then what they would produce, if they all would come into the office and they all would spend 1000 Euros, that would be a production of 100,000 Euros for your office.

Now in our calculation from these people 70% have been converted into real patients that come into the office and sit down in your chair. If they would spend 1000 Euros, you could do 70,000 Euros with these patients.

It depends on your communication skills, how many of these patients you convert into patients that accept the treatment, and that make the treatment with you and pay.

We have said in our example that you convert 70% of these patients now 70% of 70,000 would be 49,000.

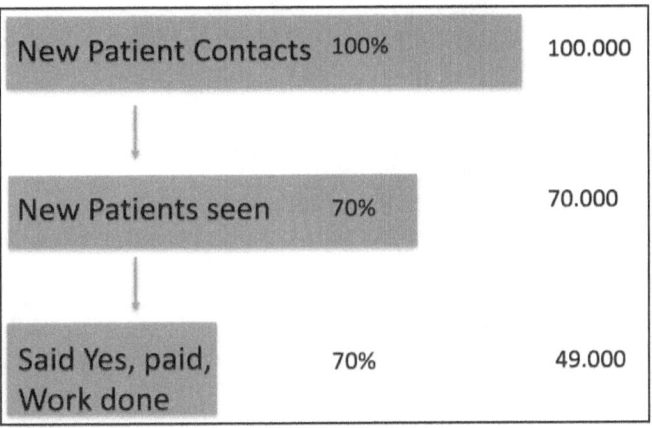

So out of 100,000 possible Euros of income, you only make 49,000 Euros of income.

Now imagine you can raise the level of your communication. So, as a consequence, the level of conversion is also higher.
Imagine that from this 100% of new patients that contact you, the front office converts 90% into patients that really come into the office and sit down in your chair. 90%.

And you with your high level of communication skill with a plan that is in the back of your mind on how to talk to the patients, you convert 90% out of the patients that sit down into patients that say yes, and the work is done and paid.

This means that from 100,000 Euros of possible income, and of all the new patients that contacted your office 90,000 possible Euros of income sit down in your chair because it's 90% of these contacts, because your front office converted 90%.

And now you convert 90% of out of these into patients that say yes, pay and you make the work.

So, in the end, you make 81,000 Euros in the same period of time, the same people have contacted your office.

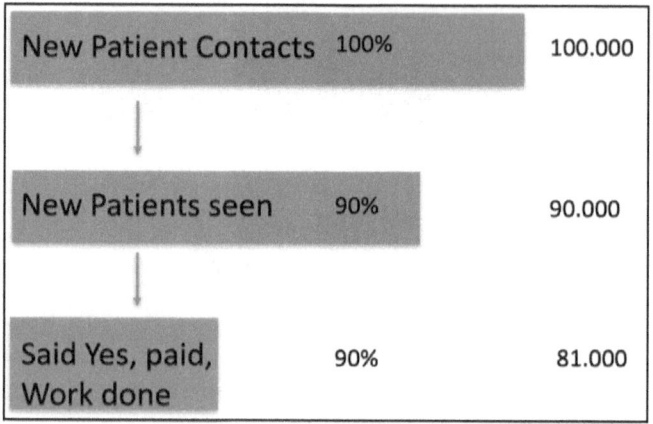

Now comparing these two levels of conversion each time: 70% or 90%. That means an increase from 49,000 Euros to 81,000 Euros.

Also, if we would talk about only 49 Euros and 81 Euros, not thousands, it's an increase always of 60% although you have only increased each step by 20% (70% to 90%).

It's extremely important to have very good communication skills to run a successful dental office.

THE BUYING HABITS

7
5 REASONS PATIENTS DON'T BUY YOUR TREATMENTS

This chapter will talk about five reasons patients don't buy your treatments and how to react to these situations, and how to make your case acceptance more successful.

<u>Reason number one.</u>

No need or low need at that moment.

You should explain to them why their health needs the treatment if they don't see the need. You need to make them see that need.

If you fail in that, then it's better to save time and move on and try maybe in a year or so. In this case follow up in half a year or a year.

But the main thing is, you need them to recognize and to see the need in that treatment.

<u>Reason number two.</u>

There is no urgency. Delay kills the sale! If they come up with "Maybe in a month, in two months, maybe later I will do that treatment", this means, that it will not happen.

It's either now or it will not happen. Show why it should be done right now. Maybe you come up with an exclusive offer, an offer you do only right now at that moment, not later. And that is why they should do it right now.

For example, you bought 10 bleaching kits for a very, very good price. And you tell the patient "Listen, I've bought 10 bleaching kits for a really good price. And I can make a good offer on the bleaching right now because there is only a limited quantity of 10. And you can get one of these for a special price", for example.

That is how you create urgency. There are ways to create urgency. Try to give them a push. It is like giving them a small reason, why they should do it right now.

So, reason number two was no urgency, you have to create urgency by exclusive offers or limited quantity. That is urgency.

Reason number three.

No desire. People usually don't buy what they need, or what is the right thing to do. Maybe *you* are convinced he needs the treatment, a periodontal treatment, for example, but the patient is not convinced. He doesn't see the need, or if he sees the need, he doesn't want it.

People do not always want what they need. They buy what they want! For example, they want the new Michael Kors™ bag or shoes or a vacation.

Do they really need that bag? These shoes, that vacation? No, they don't, they don't need that. They might need much, much more a periodontal treatment or an implant or whatever you suggest. But they don't want it.

They want that vacation. They want that Michael Kors™ bag. We don't actually need a lot of things, but we want them. We have the desire.

Here is a way you have to create the desire. With an irresistible offer, for example. Or you highlight the existing desires, they already have, and connect them to the treatment.

For example, veneers. Veneers can make the social acceptance of that person much better. They are more likable.

People want to be likable.

People want to be attractive.

People want to be confident.

People want to be socially accepted.

You have to relate your treatment, to that desire. Like a missing tooth, for example, doesn't make you very attractive, doesn't make you smile with confidence. That is why you need an implant.

Do you see the difference? They do not need an implant. They need to be socially accepted. They need to be attractive. They need to be confident.

This is what you have to aim at in your argumentation. Not that they need an implant. This is something they don't want, but they want to be socially accepted. They want to be attractive and they want to be confident.

Reason number four.

No money. They don't have the money. They don't have a budget, but who has a yearly planned budget for dentistry? People usually have a budget for a vacation, they have a budget for Christmas gifts, and so on. We have a budget for our car and so on.

But who has a budget for dentistry? Who has reserved money for dentistry? Literally nobody.

So, they don't have a budget. What's new about that? They don't have the money now available. That usually means they don't see the value in your treatment.

They don't see why that costs so much. If they don't see the value, we haven't presented the benefits of the treatment the way, that the value is higher than the price. A high value is exactly what I was addressing before. Valuable for the patients means social acceptance, it means being attractive, it means being confident.

That has a high value for the patient.

The higher the value the less the price is important. If you can create in the patient's mind the picture, that the treatment has a high value for them, then the price is not so important. They will find the money to pay for it.

And if they don't find the money, why don't you put some financing options together? Talk to your bank, if they can finance small treatments for your patients. Talk to third parties, that offer financial services to give you different options.

Reason number five.

No trust. They just don't trust you. Give them more social proof. Like testimonials, like before and afters. Have your own cases. Show them, and tell stories about the patients. "This patient was just like you. And here's how he or she looked like after the treatment. Do you see how confident she smiles? See how beautiful she is."

Attractiveness, confidence, social acceptance, social proof.

Tell them your background, make sure they know.

I did that postgraduate program,

 I graduated in this university,

I have so many years of experience all these things.

You have to make them know. How do you make them know? By telling them why you treat them, by making your hygienist tell them why she's doing the cleaning.

This gives them more reasons to trust you.

Sometimes they doubt about themselves and not you. That means they think it will not work for them. It's a waste of money. For example, the last bridge they had failed, why should it be different with you, you have to give them reasons for that, for example: "We are using so zirconium, this kind of bridges are very new and they don't fail like the ones, that have been put on you last time". "In your case, this is the correct decision", or: "in this case, we include one more pillar, one more tooth to make it more stable". This is one reason.

The other thing is, you tell them that you put them in a hygiene program to increase success in the long term. They're not left alone. "Once we do that bridge, once we do that treatment, you get into our recall-hygiene program. You come in every six months, we check, we maintain so that we make this a success in the long term. This treatment should be a success in the long term. You are not left alone. We are here to maintain this treatment."

This is the kind of message you should transmit to the patient. This is something you have to tell them. And remember:

No need, no sale.
No urgency, no sale.
No desire, no sale.
No money, no sale
and no trust, no sale.

8
3 REASONS WHY PATIENTS
BUY YOUR TREATMENTS

In this chapter, I want to talk to you about three reasons why patients buy your treatments.

If you know these three reasons you can cater to them. You promote these three reasons and make people say more "yes" to your treatment offers.

<u>Reason number one.</u>

Patients buy because of emotions, and then they justify it with logic.

They don't buy because of logic, they buy because of emotions. It feels good, it feels right. I buy it! And then they need to justify themselves for this emotional decision.

And they justify it with logic.

You have to paint the picture in their mind. You have to let them feel, they already had that treatment like veneers for example. They should feel like they smile with these beautiful teeth. Paint a picture in the mind first. And then they feel it, they have the emotions of it.

And they will decide based on these emotions, let the conversation feel right. So, if everything flows easily and it's happy and it's going well with the conversation between you and the patient, then this helps the patient to make an emotional decision.

Give them later guidance to see the urgency. Also help them to see what happens, if they do not do the treatment right now. This is also very emotional, but starting to be logic.

And then later, give them also the benefits for a logic justification. Give them all the benefits of the treatment. So that they can justify their emotional decision to make the treatment with you.

Reason number two.

Patients don't buy their way into something, but they buy a way out of something.

Not into something, what does that mean? They do not *want* the treatment. Who wants dental treatment? Nobody wants dental treatment.

They want a way out of their problem. This is what they buy. They do not buy veneers. They buy a way out of their ugly smile.

This is something very important to understand. If you understand that, you focus more on their needs, on their problems on their pain. Not physical, but psychological pain.

They have a problem, you give them the solution. The treatment is the solution to that problem. Let them be aware of their problem. Paint a picture in their mind, not only of the outcome, but also of their problem. Are there future problems involved? Are they possible with that problem that they have right now?

That is how you create a little bit of urgency and present the treatment as the solution to their pain. Their pain in the neck, just graphically speaking.

You help them to get out of this pain in the neck.

Reason number three.

Patients don't buy products or services. They buy stories.

Much more than products or services? What does that mean? That means you have to add a story to treatment.

Here are some ideas on how you add a story to a treatment.

How did you get started with that treatment? You can tell them how you did your first implant back in 1994. And since then, the techniques have evolved a lot there is a lot of new technology that has come out in the market and nowadays, we don't use the same technology you used in 1994. You paint a picture in the mind of the patient that you have a story with implantology. Or with smile design, or periodontology, orthodontic treatments, Invisalign™, or whatever.

You just have to tell the patient about your experience with it and then it becomes a story. It now is not only a treatment, but a treatment with a story, *your* story.

Another possibility would be to tell the patient why you do it. Why did you choose to do orthodontic treatments or periodontal treatments? To help patients of course. But you have to tell him then stories of people that you have treated well: "I had this patient and he wrote me a letter a few years later, thanking me for having made his smile design because he got a good job, just because of his smile".

Just a small story about a patient, who was in the same (mental) pain as your patient is now, and now got out of that pain. This story makes the patient decide more towards your treatment than towards the treatment of another dentist.

Tell (real) stories and sell (real) treatments.

PSYCHOLOGICAL RULES

9
THE PSYCHOLOGY OF SAYING YES

In this chapter, we will talk about the psychology of saying yes and you will learn the difference between persuasion and manipulation. You will learn Professor Cialdini's six principles of persuasion and how to apply them to dentistry.

Professor Robert Cialdini is a psychologist and he defined or found out the six principles of persuasion. He wrote that down in his book "Influence". It was written in the 80s and it is the basis of a lot of different psychological thinking and theories around the acceptance and the influencing and persuasion of people's choice and selection.

He found out six principles. One is reciprocity, then scarcity, authority, consistency, or commitment, then the principle of liking and the principle of consensus or social norms or social proof.

All these principles influence people in a certain way to persuade them to choose you or to choose a certain option if you use them in the right way.

Let me talk about all these principles and how to apply them to dentistry. But first, let me explain the terms Persuasion and

Manipulation.

Persuasion

This is not manipulation. Persuasion is the ability to move someone in our direction, to make him more likely to see things our way by how we present our ideas to him. Not *what* we present but *how* we present it.

It is very important to understand that psychologically, for the patient, it's not so much important, what we do what our treatment is all about, but how we present it to him, how he feels about it, how he senses this treatment or these treatment options.

If we have that in mind, then everything will be much easier for us to do. The whole presentation process will be different and we'll have a much better outcome. All goes through communication.

Our communication skills are very important for that.

Difference between Persuasion and Manipulation

Persuasion involves education, information, genuine facts, and the intention is to help. Your intention as a dentist is anyhow to help. What you do when you are talking to a patient about treatment options is to persuade him to choose that treatment that you think is the best for the patient. You are not manipulating the patient.

Manipulation involves a dishonest presentation of ideas that don't help the patient. There is no genuinity in it.

Reciprocity

The first principle would be reciprocity. It is an implied obligation. What does that mean? If somebody does something nice for us, we feel obligated or obliged to do something nice for them. That's reciprocity.

You open a door in a restaurant or open a door to a person

and this person feels sort of obliged to reopen the door for you, or to open the lift or elevator door for you later. Another example would be with friends, you pay the check in a restaurant, they feel obliged to do it the next time themselves for you.

That is reciprocity. It is nearly universal, but it does not work with self-centered people. That's the only negative thing.

It is an exchange of perceived value. If you do something, although it's not a big thing, but the other person perceives this as a really big favor, he will try to make also a big favor to you.

So, a patient usually reciprocates with loyalty, positive reviews, and referrals.

Give them eBooks, white papers about their issue if they need implants. Write some eBooks or white papers or copy and paste from somewhere and print it for them or give it as a PDF to them.

Small gifts like toothpaste, tongue-scrapers, and floss are accepted as something that can in return, reciprocate in the patient, loyalty, positive reviews, or referrals.

You can also give him special attention, move him in his schedule a little bit towards his needs. Let him know what you do for him if you just move the schedule, but he thinks that it would have been possible anyhow. If he does not perceive that you do him a favor, then he will not reciprocate. But if you let him know that you did something special for him, he will feel obliged to do something special for you. That's the principle of reciprocity.

Scarcity

The next principle is scarcity. If there are only a few available of something or it is available only for a limited time, then people are more likely to want it.

This is a psychological issue. It is a rule for most people. There are only two limiting factors.

We cannot always use scarcity:

- we cannot use it for a long period of time. Otherwise, it appears not to have any scarcity in it,
- and the second you cannot use it too often.

Time-limited offers are something that produces scarcity. So, put an added value package together. I'm not a big fan of making some discounts. I am a big fan of adding some value but charge the normal price.

For example, you may put an exam, X-ray, cleaning, and bleaching as a package. And this package is a little bit cheaper than all the components would cost together. Is that a discount? Yes, it is. It's a little bit of a discount, compared with all these four things separated. It is a discount, but in the end, you make much more money as if you would only do the exam.

Put that together and put a time limit to this offer. That's how you produce scarcity and people are more likely to want it.

Another way of time-limited offers are offers with an enhanced service.

For example, you do normally an exam, now, instead of only an exam, make an exam with oral cancer screening, but only for a limited time. You offer it for the same price you do a usual exam.

Limited time, that's the factor.

You can also make an exam and a digital smile design with it, but only for a limited time. People will want it.

Or you produce scarcity through reputation. Establish yourself as an expert in a certain field in your town, and there is only one of you in town. That's automatically scarcity.

Scarcity through scheduling for example. Produce scarcity through appointment availability although you have free appointments. When patients call in, let the front office say this week it's not possible (although you have open spaces this week), but then immediately let them say: "Let me see if I can squeeze you in".

With that you produce two things.

- First thing: you make it seem as if there is scarcity, although there is no scarcity and
- second, the front desk helps the patient out, and makes him a favor. So, you produce the feeling of reciprocity.

Or scarcity by numbers, only X number of patients get that offer or that plan. Here is just a small trick.

Imagine you think "I would so much love to make 10 veneer cases per month or 20 veneer cases per month, that would be so great". Don't announce it that way.

Announce it that this month, only 20 patients will get veneers or a veneer treatment. So people will want to be part of these 20 people or 10 people or 10 patients. That is producing scarcity by numbers.

Scarcity by date. Only until X date, or a time limited offer or you make a combination of both.

Authority

The next principle is authority. Become a trusted authority. Claim that for yourself. Be known as a dental problem solver. Dentistry is a trust-based business. You don't have to be necessarily an authority, you just have to be perceived as one.

You have also to be likable, reliable and trustworthy. You have to be seen as a likable, reliable, and trustworthy expert. Everything around you should communicate that you are the trusted expert in town. Everything! Your advertisement, your social media posts, everything should communicate you are THE trusted expert.

This authority moves people towards accepting what you say. You claim and exercise authority, every time you communicate, that increases case acceptance and builds patient loyalty.

You can also use inside of the principle of authority, third party authority to claim that the treatment that you have offered to the patient is the right choice. You say: these authorities also say or claim that with studies of prestigious universities, professors, or countries for example, Harvard University says that this treatment is the best choice in your case. That would be a third-party authority, claiming that, and this would make case acceptance much easier for your patient.

Celebrities are also a good third-party. They choose to do exactly this treatment. 'So the patient thinks: Well, if authorities do that, and they live from their smile, that's how they make their living, then it must be good'.

That's how you use authority as a psychological principle to make patients accept more your options.

Consistency

The next principle is consistency, or commitment. How does it work?

Once a public commitment to do something has been made people tend to act consistently to that commitment. If they publicly commit to something, they usually try to accomplish it.

They try, they tend to act consistently with that commitment. How can we take advantage of that? I will explain something that is not something I made up. That's a psychologically proven trick.

Instead of giving the filled-out appointment card to the patient, you give them the patient appointment, let's say Monday in two weeks at 4 pm. So instead of writing that down, in the appointment card and handing the appointment card to the patient, you hand the appointment card to the patient, blank and you give him also a pen and let him write down the appointment, the date and the time.

This makes them feel more committed to this treatment, time, and date. They write it down, they commit to the time and they do that on a psychological level. And the no-shows drop 18% without doing anything else.

Of course, you would two days or three days before the appointment, remind them about the appointment, and then one day before also and this drops the no-shows even more.

But without doing anything else, only by letting them fill out the date and hour, the no-shows drop 18% because they made a public commitment to that date and time.

Instead of being given this appointment, they wrote it down they created it in their mind, they created that appointment, it was them, they committed.

Liking

The next principle is liking. We buy from people we like much more often than we buy from people we don't like. Well, that's logical, I know.

But how can we be likable for our patients, to make them buy from us more than from other dentists?

Likability is strongly based on how similar they are to us or we are to them. Find a commonality with this patient, for example, the town where you were born, the school you went to, the high school you went to, the University you went to, also the cultural level, hobbies, interests. For example, you married a venezuelan woman, like I did, my beautiful wife, and the patient also married a hispanic woman.

These are certainly commonalities you have with a patient. Or both of you have children, or you are fans of a certain soccer team or baseball team, or whatever.

All these things you have to find out in the smalltalk at the beginning of the appointment, and then bring that to the surface during the presentation.

Make him see that you are similar to him. You get a positive connection also through genuine compliments, once one has found commonalities. But this works only if it is really true and you praise them when they deserve it. Everybody likes a compliment.

I like your dress or how you dress or wow you look like a person that really is into fashion or something like that.

Or: wow, this mouth is really well treated or well taken care of, and it's an expert who says that. The patient feels much better with you. He likes you a lot. Everybody does.

Then listen to your patients. If you show honest interest when they are speaking and you are present with your mind, too, then they like you more.

Likability has nothing to do with the technical aspects of dentistry. Nothing to do with your technical ability, with your skills, technical and clinical skills, and knowledge.

If people like you, they will buy from you much more than if they don't like you. Nothing to do with your skills.

Consensus

The last principle is the consensus or social norms or social proof.

People want to follow what those around them, who are similar to them, are already doing. This means we look a lot on what others do because we want to feel part of the group.

In this case, what helps are reviews. Manage them! If the patient sees a lot of reviews on your website or in Google Places or Yelp, and positive reviews of course, then that's good for you because that is social proof.

Thank patients who give you good reviews and ask patients to make reviews for you.

This is our most popular choice

If you say, for example, this treatment is the most popular choice, most of the people
- use this here or
- choose this treatment,
- choose this type of implant
- choose this type of veneers,
- choose not to make six but 10 veneers,

this is what most people choose in our office, then the patient would be more likely to choose exactly that and not something else.

Proven psychologically (Cialdini): the number of patients who say yes raises 20% than if you don't say this is the most popular choice.

Similar results are achieved with the sentence: "This is increasing in popularity". So, this treatment choice is increasing in popularity among our patients, that makes also 20% more say yes to that treatment, than if you would not say that.

10
CREATE IDEAL ACCEPTANCE CONDITIONS

In this chapter, we want to talk about how to create ideal acceptance conditions. And you will learn the different strategies to make it easier for the patient to say yes, and how to build a solid basis for a successful case presentation conversation.

The three main reasons why patients don't buy the treatments.

One, and the most important one, is the lack of **trust**.
- They don't trust you.
- They don't trust what you say.
- They don't trust whether or not you are the right person to do the treatment.
- They don't trust that you are clinically skilled for that.

There is obviously no established rapport between you and the patient.

Rapport building is made first, inside of the small talk before the real conversation and second, throughout the questions you are making and how your body language and your tonality react to the patient while you are making these questions.

These two things help you to establish rapport.

The second reason is that it is not a **priority** for them. The treatment that you're now offering or the condition they are just now in are not priorities for them.

Their priorities are much more like this: for example, to go on vacations, to buy a new car, and similar things. But let's be honest: who has dentistry as a priority except for dentists and hygienists?

No "crisis" has been created in his mind, he does not think this is so important. For you, it's important to make the patient see that it's very important to get this fixed. Only then you can make a good sale of your treatment.

The third reason is, that there is no sense of **urgency**.

Maybe they trust you. Maybe they think, "yes, it's a priority". But for them, it's not urgent. In their mind, we can make that in a few months. If it doesn't hurt, it doesn't look too bad, it can wait. That's what they usually think.

The number one reason we said it was no trust, they don't trust you. You have to build trust. You can do that before they even come to your office, by branding yourself.

Let's see the other reasons also, while money is only a reason for less than a third of the patients (source: Spear Education 2017). Spear Education made a survey in 2017. They found out the reasons why patients don't buy the treatments. And there we see that only 31% said they didn't have the money. That does not mean that they won't buy. If you give these patients, these 31% of patients, good payment options, financial options, then you can convert most of them into patients that will do the treatment.

Other reasons are "my schedule was too busy" or "I didn't have time", which is the same thing. You have to adapt to the time of the timeframes of the patients.

"I was afraid of the procedure". That's nearly 20% of the people said they were afraid.

"Found the resources I was given were confusing" (14%), these patients were confused. Here, the communication of the dentist was not clear enough.

"I didn't want to proceed to do the procedure" = 14%, but why they didn't want to do the procedure? Who knows.

"Insurance didn't cover it". 5% only.

"I didn't see how the procedure would benefit me"(5%). Here again, the communication skills of the dentist were not good enough.

That's why it's so important to create skills in communication and in sales, presenting, closing, and so on.

We need to understand one thing of the patients before they come to the office, we need to know what they are thinking. People think very much alike.

Lifestyle

And lifestyle is a big issue for a lot of patients. Bleaching Veneers, Smile Makeovers, smile design, all this enhances your lifestyle. Like a beautiful car. Like fashion. It enhances your lifestyle.

Why is that so important? Because people will pay or find a way to get the money for what they want, long before they pay for what they need.

They want lifestyle enhancement. That's what they want. Here is an example: how many pairs of shoes does a woman need? How many does she really have? How many Michael Kors™ bags does a woman really need? How many does she really want?

And they will find the money to pay although they don't need it. They want it. They find a way to pay for it. They want lifestyle enhancement. You have to understand this, you have to create an atmosphere of lifestyle enhancement so that they see the value of having a better lifestyle with that treatment that you will provide to them.

It's very true that when it comes to utility, people usually want the cheap but when it comes to lifestyle, they want the best (Fred

Joyal). So here is the key.

For example, socks. There are a lot of people that think that socks are a utility. They want the cheap in the utility. They don't have to be Gucci™ socks. But when it comes to lifestyle, for example, the suit they buy, then they want to have a Boss™ suit or a Gucci™ suit or similar brands. In their lifestyle they spend money, but in socks, they might want to save money.

If the patient sees you as a utility, then he is not in a position that he wants to spend money on you, or more money than with other dentists.

If you can explain to the patient that you, instead of just a utility, are a lifestyle enhancer, then most probably they will want to be treated by the best professional for this lifestyle enhancement.

And, of course you have to transmit the idea or the perception that you are one of the best or even the best professional to do that.

Don't be cheap. That's a very important issue. If you are cheap, you run under "utility", you are not a lifestyle enhancement, you are not the best.

Value
Another thing, why people spend money or why people buy or why people are more likely to say yes is that they need to perceive value. You don't have to sell your price you don't have to justify your price.

Price is not the major driving factor in purchasing decisions. You have to make a value proposition for your patients.

Starbucks took people from complaining about paying 50 cents for a cup of coffee to gladly paying €3 or more and stand in a line to do that, how do they do it?

They created an atmosphere that added value to the product which is a coffee. You need to create an atmosphere that adds value to your treatments.

You can also put packages together because patients want value for their money. How do you create value or the perception of value?

Try to set your fee as a package deal and show the true value of what you offer.

Instead of saying how much whitening is, for example, €525, that sounds too much. You have to put it as a package. And then by adding value €525 don't look too much.

```
Our Fläsh Procedure Fee includes:
  –  Free plaque removal on the day of Bleaching    – 40€
  –  Whitening Procedure                            - 760€
  –  Custom-fitted trays                            - 250 €
  –  Post care Take-Home Whitening Gel              - 150 €

Whitening Package: €525!
Valued at €1,200
```

You say for example: our Fläsh™ (a leading whitening brand in Europe) procedure fee includes first a free plaque removal on the day of bleaching, that's not a cleaning. It's only that you brush the teeth. That has a value of €40. You say "well I do that for free". I understand that. Imagine if a patient would come into your office and said: "listen, I just want you to clean my teeth, not a dental cleaning, but only go over my teeth with a little bit of Polish powder and the rotation brush, and I will go to your competitor to make the bleaching". How much would you charge? Put a number on it. In my example case, it's €40.

Then the whitening procedure per se. You put a price on that which is in this case, an example case, €760 and then you do custom-fitted trays, although it is an in-office whitening, you do also custom-fitted trays for the touch-ups later in half a year or one year. You include that into the procedure. You might say again "well, I do that for free, too". Imagine again, a patient comes and says "Listen, I want you to make trays for me. I will do the bleaching with another dentist". How much would you charge for these? Put that on the list.

And then post care take-home whitening gel, which means either whitening gel or post-care desensitizing gel. How much would you charge if the patient only would like to have that?

Put a price on it and then you add up all these things that you do for the patient inside of the bleaching procedure. And then the patient sees a value, an overall value. This overall value, added all together, would be 1200 Euros. But you are offering all this for only €525.

Now, it looks much cheaper than if you only say the price. That is a value offer, a package deal.

Menus

Offer menu options. If you calculate the possibilities from the menu, they offer over 10,000 different variations of coffee drinks available in any Starbucks.

You can also offer different options to the patient and he just chooses, for example, in bleaching you can have a menu set up with your price at the end. At least three options.

	Type		Product	Method	Procedure includes	Price
In- Office			with lamp	one session in the office about 1 hour	-Plaque removal -Fläsh procedure 32% -Trays -Post-treatment	X €
Combined			combined lamp and take-home	1 hour in-office + 1 week at home	-Plaque removal -Fläsh procedure 6% -Trays -Post-treatment -Take-home gel	X €
Take-Home			individual tray	2 weeks at home	-Plaque removal -Trays -Take-home gel	X €

First option: you make a whitening with a lamp in one session in the office in about one hour. Inside of the procedure you include plaque removal, the Fläsh™ procedure, in this case it's the Fläsh™ system with 32% of hydrogen peroxide. Trays and post-treatment with desensitizing gel for example, and this package has the value of x Euros.

You can also make a combined bleaching with a lamp and a take-home option. It's one hour in the office and one week at home. You make a procedure that includes plaque removal, the Fläsh™ procedure but not with 32% hydrogen peroxide, but with only 6% hydrogen peroxide to reduce to zero the possible sensitivities. But because it's not so strong, the patient has to bleach at home to get to a good level of white. Then you include the trays inside of this procedure, the post-treatment with desensitizing gel, and the take-home gel and this has another price than the first option.

And the third option is a take-home whitening. You make individual trays, it's two weeks at home every night and you include the plaque removal, the trays, and the take-home gel. And that's another price.

This is the bleaching menu that you can put in your office and the patient decides. In any case you sell a whitening. The difference is *what* kind of whitening you will sell.

What about other treatments, implants for example? Also here you can have three different types of implants and offer three different options to the patient.

For example, in our office, we differentiate between a Standard implant, a Professional implant, and a Luxury implant. This would be like an economy class, business class, and first class in an airline. All are in the same plane and all get from A to B.

choose YOUR IMPLANT	STANDARD € implant + met.-cer. crown	PROFESSIONAL € implant + met.-cer. crown	LUXURY € implant + met.-cer. crown
KEY FEATURES			
Origin of the Implant	Corea	European Union	European Union
ISO and CE - Certificates	✓	✓	✓
Guarante - all components	4 years	7 years	7 years
Scientific background	-	✓	✓
CAD-CAM components	-	✓	✓
> 30 years research	-	-	✓
CROWNS			
Dental Lab	European Union	European Union	European Union
High Esthetic Crown	-	✓	✓
UPGRADES			
Zirconium-Ceramic Crown	+ 150 €	+ 150 €	+ 150 €

What does that mean? It includes the implant and the crown. All prosthetic parts and surgical parts. What's the difference?

The price is different. And what makes the price different? You make a menu and you show to the patient what is different in all these options.

For example, in this case, the first option is the standard option. The origin of the implant is from Korea. In the professional and luxury option, it's from the European Union. All three have ISO and CE certificates. There is a guarantee difference between these three options. 4 years for the standard option 7 years for the professional option and 7 to 10 years for the luxury option.

The different implant systems have different scientific backgrounds. One of the implants, the luxury one, has more than 30 years of research. And that's a very stable thing.

The crowns are all made in the European Community. But the first crown (standard option) is made in a small lab around the corner, but the other two options have the crown from a more expensive lab. In all the options, you can upgrade to a zirconium-ceramic crown for 150 Euros more.

That's the menu for implants. You can do that for nearly every treatment. For example, periodontal treatment. With or without laser assisting. Laser-assisted periodontal treatment, LAPT, there you already have different options.

Cleanings: prophylaxis or basic cleaning, you have different options. Show these options. Make menus and show the patient different options for the different treatments.

Powerpoints

The power of PowerPoints. Imagine the patient sits down in your reception area and you have a big screen showing PowerPoints of before and afters of your own cases and project them in the reception hall and all the dental units. He passes from the reception area to the chair sits down in the chair before you come he also sees all these cases before and after.

Merchandise your office.

Imagine how an old office looks like. All these pictures of extraction instruments and surgical appliances, historical drawings, anatomy posters. You want to avoid exactly this.

But you also want to avoid pictures, that have nothing to do with what you do and offer. What are you, a travel agency that you have the Taj Mahal or a poster of the Eiffel Tower?

What are you really selling? You are selling smiles and you have to merchandise your office for that. You have to show beautiful smiles, happy people and this, unconsciously gets into the mind of the patient. All these smiles unconsciously help the patient to decide to enhance his smile. Merchandise your office with smiling and happy people, that represent exactly the kind of patient, that you want to attract to the office.

Build Trust

Remember the number one reason for patients not to buy? It was a lack of trust. Build trust, be credible. How well are *your* teeth bleached? Do you have beautiful teeth? If you don't have beautiful teeth, you have yellowish teeth and they are cracked and crowded, how can you think that the patient will be thinking of making a smile-design or a smile make-over with you, if *you* don't do it for yourself. Enhance your credibility with that.

Do it also with your whole staff. Everybody in your office, even the cleaning lady, should have really beautiful teeth. That pushes up your credibility.

To build trust, you can also publish in local or national newspapers and magazines. You can write articles in newspapers and journals about bleaching. If nobody wants to publish something about you, you can do it in free press releases (www.free-press-release.com).

From there, you can even take ideas for your publications.

Brand yourself.

Branding is a big issue. And there will be a whole book on that, too. Branding is the best long-term strategy for success. A polished and more professional look is a way to create a unique identity for your dental office. For you and your dental office. People should connect your office with strong and positive emotions. That's branding.

Branding is what people think about you. How do you want people to think about you? How do you want people to talk about you? Be like that, behave like that.

Branding is promising. Consistency makes your office recognizable. You have to have a strong web presence, that builds trust. And it should be beautiful.

That's our website for example. These are images from Valencia. We show these pictures because part of our business comes from dental tourism from Northern European Countries.

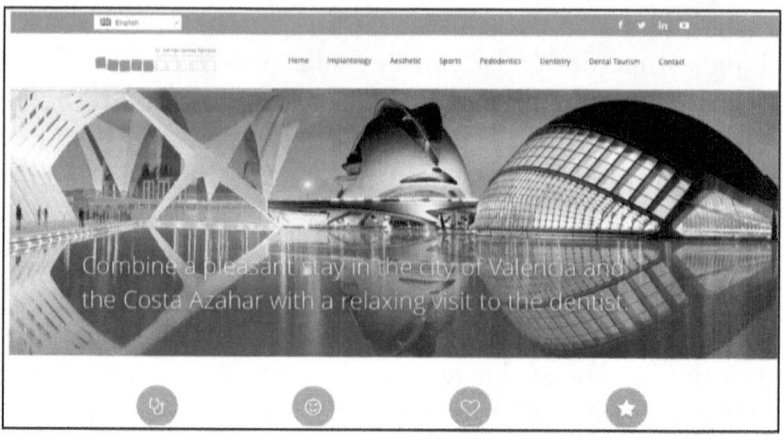

Show where you are, who you are, what you do, and all this in a beautiful way.

Then do info events, open doors events, to build trust to build credibility. Offer information evenings for persons who are interested in white or healthy teeth, or implants.

Also hire a publicist to build trust. A publicist is a person, usually a journalist, that has connections with the media, press, radio, television, local television, national television, and who makes you appear news-worthy. And that's why you are invited to these media.

You don't pay the media to be there, to appear in them. That would be another way to go. But the media call you because this guy made them aware of you and of the message that you want to deliver.

In my case, for example, on local radio. They get you into the media for free. You don't pay the media you pay this guy, which is the same but in the end, the media will not sell you as somebody who paid this message, but somebody who is newsworthy, so your credibility boosts up.

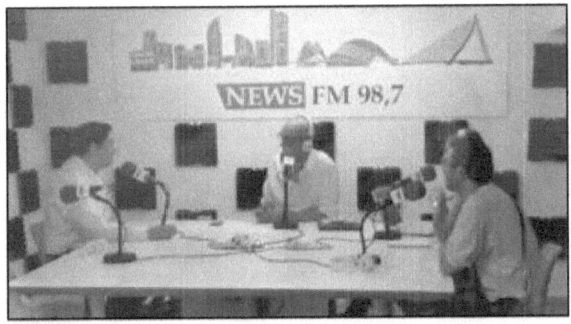

Then on TV, also local TV in Valencia.

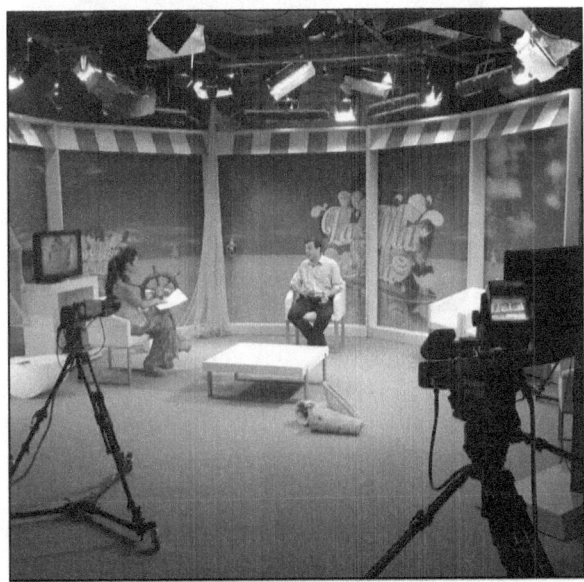

Or you can make your own Extreme Makeover™ as Dr. Bill Dorfman did. Well, he did not do his own Extreme Makeover™ he *was* the dentist of Extreme Makeover™.

You can just copy him. You can do the same but on a local TV channel or if nobody wants to publish that, publish it on YouTube.

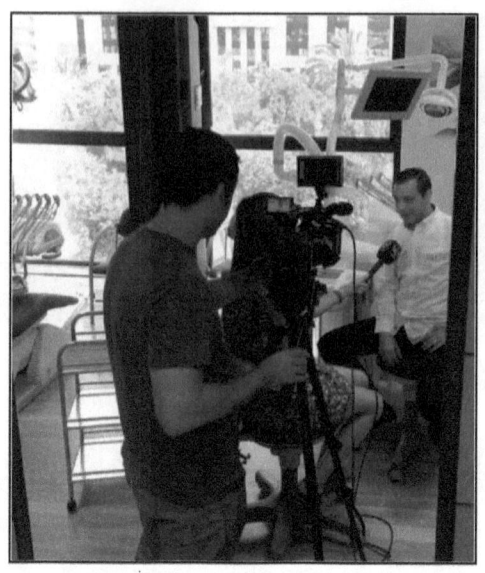

Search a
- plastic surgeon in your town,
- and an ophthalmologist,
- a personal trainer,
- a dietician,
- a hairstylist,
- a makeup specialist,
- and a personal stylist that helps people to dress better.

Then you have put your own local team together. Transform cases together. It's professionally rewarding and fun.

You also have to get strong in social media to be able to build trust. People before they call you, they look you up. If you are strong on social media, your reputation is already good and your trust goes up.

Social media marketing main goals are:
- to increase your reputation
- to get more and or better patients (I prefer better patients than more patients),

- to drive traffic to your website,
- to collect emails from people who are interested in you
- to get phone calls for appointments.

You can also blog or vlog every week or every month. Do a video every month, do a blog every month to build trust, to build credibility.

<u>The importance of being liked</u>
There is nothing so important than to be likable. Have you ever *not* bought something because you didn't like the salesperson? Of course! You wanted to buy something, went to the store and you didn't like the salesperson, you didn't buy. You went to another store you bought it there.
The same thing happens here in dentistry.
Have you ever bought with a final decision because you like the person? Imagine you were indecisive of whether to buy or not to buy. And you really like the person that sells you the item that you maybe want to buy. Then you maybe will buy, but if people dislike you, you have no chance.
Liking won't make them buy, but it does make it possible.

We have different stages or possibilities in the buying decision of a patient. Here are several examples:

Imagine, they are keen on the treatment you offer.
If they like you, it's sold.
If they don't like you, it's probably not sold although they wanted it, and although they're keen on it.

Imagine, they have not yet decided whether or not to buy the treatment, but they're a little bit in favor of it.
If they like you, it's very likely for them to buy.
If they don't like you, it's very unlikely for them to buy.

Imagine, they have not yet decided whether or not to buy the

treatment, but they're a little bit against it, marginally against it.
If they like you, you still can make them buy the treatment.
But if they don't like you, it's not going to happen.

Imagine they don't want it or are against buying it (but imagine it is a necessary treatment, that – if not done – would worsen the situation or even threaten the patient's health).
If they then like you, you have a small possibility to sell the treatment.
If they don't like you, there's not a hope to sell that treatment.

Most of the patients haven't decided yet. And you can turn them around by being likable.

In another chapter I describe some ways to be likable.

11
PRE-SUASION PRINCIPLES

In this chapter, we will talk about pre-suasion principles. This means how to put people previously in a mood to say yes to your treatment. You will see pre-suasion in different situations and how to apply them to dentistry.

Pre-suasion is based on Professor Dr. Robert Cialdini. He is a psychologist. And he wrote a book just recently, that is called "pre-suasion". He has also written a book in the 80s that is called "influence".

Pre-suasion is the process of arranging for a patient to agree to your offer *before* he encounters it. Before you make the offer, you already have arranged the patient to agree.

That is not a magical trick, that is established science and it follows certain rules of psychology.

It is about what you say and do immediately before you deliver your message. You prepare the ground first. This is unperceived by the patient 100% of the times, scientifically proven. They don't know they are influenced just before they are offered a treatment. Because they don't know they are influenced, they don't get it. Then they make the decision very unconsciously, of accepting your treatment.

Let me explain to you several things that are pre-suading people and how to apply them to dentistry. It flies under the radar, people just don't detect it. Because their defense is low when you apply pre-suasion, as it is before the actual offer.

Usually when you make an offer, when you make a presentation, when you explain the treatment, people put on defenses. But *before* that, if you do something or say something or draw the attention or put a seed into the mind before you start the presentation, the defenses of the patient are low at that moment, and you will have direct access to his mind.

Pre-suasion

The choices that we make are more related to what is in our top-of-mind at that moment. When you do some pre-suasion, you do something that causes the patient to have a positive state of mind towards the idea or the concept of your (following) message.

If you want to sell flowers, you put the idea of spring and beautiful landscapes upfront. You can mention flowers when you don't need to mention flowers, people are already open to the concept of flowers. At that moment, you cause in the patient to have a positive state of mind towards the idea or the concept of your message, of your treatment *before* you deliver the message or before you offer the treatment.

A communicator can put us in mind of a particular concept, for example, a concept in dentistry would be:
fixed versus removable, in this example the concept would be "fixed". You can put the patient into a mode of fixed solutions. Another example would be metal-free or white aesthetics, or any strength of a treatment, for example high quality.

If we mention things related to these examples before the

presentation, then we would channel the patient's mind to think about that as a more important factor in his choice.

You plant the seed immediately before you offer a smile make-over because the patient is thinking about how white is so beautiful.

Also, a background picture influences decisions. Robert Cialdini describes an example that is very easy to understand. There is an online marketer for a factory that sells furniture. They sell all sorts of furniture high quality and expensive, but also cheap types. They sell that online.

They made an experiment that half of the people that came to their website, and they didn't know who was the person that came to the website, were directed to the same website, but with a background of nice clouds. The idea of comfort was given to them, being comfortable, being like in the cloud when you sit down on a very comfortable sofa. This gives you the feeling of being seated on a cloud.

The other half was directed to the same website but as background picture they had coins, money, change.

The people that were directed to the clouds as background were much more interested in looking up very comfortable furniture. Compared to the half of the people that were directed to the coins and money, they were more interested in looking up much more the cheap furniture.

They made this experiment with so many people that it was very significant. This background picture, conditioned the mind to think about a feature, the feature was either saving money, or it was comfort and then their interest was channeled.

You can do that in your office, too. You need to recognize what the central element of your message is. For example, fixed for implants, or metal free white for Veneers and smile make-overs.

What is the benefit of a treatment that would make it wise for the patient to accept the offer? And then go to the moment before you deliver the offer and draw the patient's attention to this idea.

By shifting the patient's attention towards a particular concept or idea, we not only shift their attention, but we also shift who they are at that moment.

If I shift your attention towards romance, I can make you a romantic.

If I shift your attention towards price, I can make you a cost-orientated buyer.

If I shift your attention towards quality, I can make you a quality-focused purchaser.

Environment

An expensive high-quality environment channels the mind to make more expensive and high-quality choices. It doubles the possibility, according to the psychological science described by Cialdini. The environment is one of the pre-suasion situations. Pictures, posters, pictures on screens. We have veneers, implants, smile design, high-quality things, your appointment cards showing a smile, preconditions the people.

"What is focal is causal" - Phenomenon

Another situation of pre-suasion is the "what is focal is causal". Where I focus on is the cause of the situation. Although there is no causal relation for us, in our subconscious mind, we think, it's related.

In reality it's not, but we think what we are paying attention to normally in our environment, we perceive as the cause of what is going on. That was shown in psychological experiments.

In American football games, for example, some players were highlighted in their dresses, and the referees were always focusing on them. Whenever there was a bad situation, most of the time they thought these guys were the cause of that bad situation and punished them. So, what we are paying attention to normally in our environment, we perceive as the cause of what is going on.

Draw the attention to a feature, a veneer or implant in a picture when you show the picture or when you show a before and after picture, you send the patient's attention to a certain thing and he believes that it is the cause of the whole beauty or that the patient is so happy.

<u>They should pre-own it</u>

Another situation is the pre-owning. You paint the picture in their mind already owning a certain treatment.

A lot of car salespeople make that. They make you picture yourself in the Mercedes™ driving around. And this helps them to sell that Mercedes™.

You paint a picture in the mind of the patient owning a certain treatment. They will then prioritize this one above an alternative treatment.

The patient comes in and before you even present anything you just mention. "Ah, today I'm so happy (you show happiness). A patient just walked out with a beautiful new smile (you mention beauty) with veneers. Stunning. She was so thankful and so happy (his mind gets: thankful, happy, happiness, beautiful, veneers).

What do you think the patient will think right now about all the things? He will relate happiness and beauty to veneers, unconsciously.

Then, if you say: in your case, we would be able to do a bonding, that means fillings in the front, or veneers. The patient is already pre-sold on veneers, because just when the patient walked in you pre-conditioned his mind, you pictured it. He saw in his mind the patient walking out with the veneers and said thought, that it would be nice if he would also have veneers.

You pre-sold the patient on that.

The Need to Closure

The next pre-suasion situation is the need to closure. Everybody needs to close or solve a mystery.

You open a mystery: why are we as an office or me as a dentist perceived as the top implantology office in town? Now people are paying more attention to what you say next, compared to if you just say it without this opening question.

You have to make a question out of the message that you want to deliver. If you just deliver the message, it can go in one ear and out the other ear. They don't pay attention to it. If you make it as a mystery, why do you think we are perceived as the top implantology clinic in town? They ask themselves.. why? And then you deliver your message like

- your experience,
- your continuous education in very important academies or universities,
- and all the advantages you have in modern equipment and all these things.

Now he gets the message. He understands why your quality is so high. Why? Maybe because

- we use the highest quality implants
- we have a highly trained team

The patient understands that because he focuses now, because he wants to solve the mystery why you are perceived as the top office in veneers or smile design, why you?

Notice, that you don't claim, that you are the best or that you do this or that. No, you ask: why are we perceived as the top office in town for this or that? And then he starts to listen. After that, you say we do this, this and that, and he gets the message. Now the attention is drawn to your next message. That's the trick.

Pre-question

As people want the questions to be solved, also pre-questions are another different way, and that is another situation of presuasion.

One question at the beginning focuses the new patient on the positive aspects of you or your office. For example, before you even start discussing anything with the patient, he is already open-minded if you ask him one question. With this question, he can already be put in a positive attitude towards you.

How can you do that? You say:

- why did you choose us today? Or
- what made us interesting for you to choose us?

What is he now thinking? He's thinking about the positive things that made him call you. That is already pre-selling him on you.

What made us interesting for you to choose us? That's a very good question. Some pre-questions will help people to decide to do something. There was an experiment that people went up to other people and asked them to help them in a survey. Only 29% agreed to help them in that survey. The same people went to other people asking them a pre-question. The question was:

Do you consider yourself a helpful person?

And people usually think: yeah, of course, I'm helpful.

And then they asked them to help them in a survey. 77.3% agreed to help them in the survey.

Do you see how it boosts up? So, pre-questions preconditioned the mind to do something or to think about something that you want to sell or do later.

Do you consider yourself a quality-oriented person?, for

example. You focus the mind of the patient towards quality.

Do you consider yourself a beauty-oriented person? You pre-condition the mind of the patient to beauty.

Do you consider yourself a comfort-oriented person? You can focus the mind of the patient towards comfort.

Do you consider yourself a stability-oriented person? In a person that has dentures that are not very stable, that makes him immediately think about stability and fixed solutions.

And then you offer them different options and they will choose unconsciously the stability-oriented option (following our last example).

Not 100% of the people not 100% of the time, but you can get much more patients do what you want them to do.

THE PROCESSES

12
THE CLOSING SEQUENCE

In this chapter, we will talk about the closing sequence. That means the steps we are going to do from the beginning until the end of the close.

We will learn what is the aim of the sequence is. You will get to know the steps and have a structure you can always follow. You will have a clear structure in your mind and you follow this red line, from the beginning to the end, so that everything makes sense what you do.

What's the aim of the closing sequence? The final aim of the closing process is to create certainty. Certainty in an uncertain world.

The patient is uncertain about whether or not he should do a treatment. Whether or not he should spend money, he should undergo a, sometimes, painful surgery.

You have to convert this uncertainty in certainty. This is the aim of the closing sequence. Uncertainty becomes certainty and then the patient moves forward.

Step 1 – Immediate Control

The first step is, you have to get immediate control of the situation. How? You have to show you are an expert, make your homework on the patient. That means you have to have information on the patient, he has to like you. He only likes you if you know a lot of things about the patient and let him speak.

Brand yourself right. You can have done that with your marketing, with your social media, with Your videos. But don't expect that everybody has seen your videos, don't expect that everybody has seen your Instagram or your Facebook account and knows everything you have posted. Not everybody knows that.

In the conversation at the beginning, you just, by the way, mention how great your experiences with this treatment is. How many patients you have done with this treatment "and the best thing is…" you just tell in a story about a patient who just came in last week with exactly that problem, very similar to the problem the patient has now, and how happy he was later.

And then you, by the way mention the hundreds and hundreds of patients in the last 20 years that you have done in this kind of treatment.

You have told the patient, I am doing this kind of treatment for 20 years and have been trained here or there. Or you can explain to him dozens of patients that you have done since you made the post-graduate continuing education course in for example Dubai, with the Mastery Academy™ or something like that.

You have to brand yourself right. And only with that, the patient sees you as an expert. I know he is already in the office, I know he thinks you are good, otherwise, he would not be there.

But you have to get a higher level of confidence. So that the patient sees you in the light you want him to see you.

That is very important. So, here you already start to build rapport. Later in step three, you build more rapport.

Your success depends on your ability to interact with others. This first step is a small talk step. In this small talk, you just let him know a lot about you. Also, this is the only time where you are allowed to talk about you and your team and your experience.

Your success depends on the ability to interact with others. So, make communication courses, that is very important, and positively influence them. Positive because you are sure this treatment is the correct one for them. And if you do that treatment that would be the best thing ever for them, then it's positive for them.

Step 2 – Gather Information

The second step would be to gather information. In that step, which is part of a patient communication book, you have to find out several things. You have to ask smart questions to find out the pain points of the patient, the needs of the patient, and if he is financially qualified, if he can afford it.

You don't need 100 reasons for a patient to buy your treatment. You have to find out which ones are the right ones that he needs to know.

Let them make 80% of the talk. You just ask questions and if there is something that is not clear enough, you say: "tell me more about that". You need information to determine if your patient can afford the treatment and if it is in his best interest to get that treatment. Important is the tonality of your questions.

Do it in an interested way, as if you were completely interested in the patient and empathetic. Honesty, curiosity, tonality, and body language, build rapport with the patient.

If he starts to talk about other things not relevant for you, don't interrupt him. Wait until he has finished speaking, but you have to redirect the conversation. So, don't go more into this unnecessary direction because you lose time, and time is money in the dental office. But you don't interrupt the patient, and your body language should not show that he's going in the wrong direction. You are interested, remember?

You have to be curious, honestly curious. But once he stopped doing it, redirect him again back to what is important for his treatment. What he is running away from, what he doesn't like of his situation, and what he needs.

Don't be disrespectful. You say: "That is interesting. It sounds like you've had a great time with your grandchildren last weekend, very nice". So, and then you redirect. "By the way, let me ask you a question….." and then you ask your next question to find out the needs.

If he asks you whether or not you like XY, and you don't. For example, "do you like soccer?"

And imagine you don't like soccer.

Don't say: "No, I don't like soccer." Maybe he likes soccer. You say: "I wish I had more time to get more into soccer, but I don't have time so I'm not so into it right now".

This respects his possible passion for that sport and it does not get you into a bad light because you don't like it. And you continue with

"By the way…", and then your next question from your side in that gathering-information-process.

"By the way, how do you like the color of your teeth"

Step 3 – Build rapport

The third step is to build rapport. While you ask the questions, he has to feel that your body language and your tonality are completely focused on him, not on you, on him. And that you are very interested in helping him.

Build trust, show empathy through tonality and your body

language. But they need to like you also, so stop trying to be interesting yourself, people like you, if you show interest in them. People like people that are interested in them, and let them talk and who appreciate the good things of this person

Nobody gets that enough times in his life. You cater to that, and he likes you. He likes you more than another dentist, where he did also go to find out about the prices and the treatment. You have to be different.

Show a huge interest in your patient. That is the trick.

The aim of building rapport is that the patient has to like you and see you as a highly competent professional in general. As someone who knows the treatment inside and out and is passionate about its value.

You have to be likable. You have to be very competent and professional and you have to be passionate.

You need to manage your emotional and physical state. If you are in a bad mood, that's not good. Get that away from you. Be positive in front of a patient. You have to be enthusiastic and positive. Always!

You have to brighten the patient's day. People like to be around other people that brighten up their days. Everybody likes that. Think about one of your friends that is always happy, always smiling, always lifting up everybody, always positive, always enthusiastic. Of course, you like to be around him, you like to invite him to dinner, you like to spend weekend-barbecue-time with this kind of friend.

Of course, everybody likes to be around people that are positive, enthusiastic, and brighten up their days. And on top, if these people are interested or show genuine interest in you, perfect, then a big rapport is made.

And this rapport is very important. For the closing.

You have to lift everybody. Your job is to raise the patient up into a state of happiness and empowerment. If he is happy and empowered the close is easier.

Step 4 – Transition

And then you make the transition. You transition into your presentation. You have all the information you need, and you know what's right for the patient. You have to transition in a way like:

here is what we can do for you or
here is what we will do for you.

But in other words. Much better would be:

"Based on what you have said to me, or
based on everything you have told me,

this is the perfect solution for you.
Let me tell you why".

That is the transition. And then you start to present.

Step 5 - Presentation

That is the fifth step, the presentation. Why the advantages of your treatment solution (the WHY is more important), are going to solve the problems of the patient. So, you have seen the problems, you have gathered the problems (step 2), you have written them down, and then you say, this will solve that problem.

And don't shoot all your guns yet, you need to have some arguments, some advantages reserved for when he starts to object, then you can put out more things.

If you have shut all your guns and he makes an objection, there's nothing left for you. You cannot shoot another advantage. Presentation techniques are part of a different book, but you need to know, that you don't shoot all your guns in your presentation.

Step 6 – Wrap up your Recommendation

Then the sixth step is to wrap up your recommendation. You have to add more value to your proposal. You make the presentation and you say there's a guarantee, or so many years of guarantee because we use this highly advanced Swiss material. You state as a reason your background and credibility with that treatment.

Here it comes again, what you started in the first step. You have made this treatment like 200 times and virtually all the patients are really happy.

Virtually. Not all patients are really happy. Maybe one or two are not happy, but "virtually all" is correct. So, you don´t lie, although some patients might not be completely happy.

You can show before and afters then, that wraps up the recommendation. And patient testimonials about that treatment, like this you can lift the value so that the price that you say to the patient seems to be low.

The patients buy into the reasons of *why* you are doing something much more than *what* it is what you do.

They don't care about what it is what you do. We put some veneers on the teeth. No, this is not a reason to buy for the patients.

Why are you doing that? You want to make for example a smile beautiful and even, that is why we do the veneers.

It's not about explaining to him the sequence of the treatment. It's about explaining to him why we do that? The WHY lifts the value.

We will put some veneers on your teeth (why) because this helps us to enlarge this tooth and wow, that is beautiful. That is exactly why we're doing it. Now it has another value.

Before that, it was just a piece of information on what steps you will do for the patient.

The what is what steps you will do **with** the patient.

The why is why you are doing it **for** the patient.

You understand the difference.

Then summarize everything you told him and move to the next step which is the close.

Step 7 – Ask for the Order

You ask for the order, the close, that is the seventh step.

Ask for what you want. What do you want to do? Well, you want to make the treatment. You ask, let me make the treatment.

In other words, of course, you use one of these techniques that I have shown you, one of the 10 closing techniques.

If you Don't ask. You don't get it.

Step 8 – First Objection

And then the eighth step is your first objection.

The real sales process doesn't start until the patient says no. Now the real sales process starts. Until then, it was easy. And if he doesn't have any objection, it's fluid.

Here comes the real skill of selling. When the patient says no, or objects, your job is to reframe this objection, until the no becomes a yes.

Objection handling techniques are described in a previous chapter. Your first objection, maybe" I get back to you", "I don't know", "let me think it over", the uncertainty is strong.

Remember what your aim is. Your aim is to create certainty. Obviously, this certainty has not been created and has not been reached. So, you need to go back again and try to build up this certainty.

With a deflection technique and looping, for example:

"I hear or I see what you are saying.
- But does the idea make sense to you?
- Do you like the idea?
- Do you see what I see?"

No,

then "why not? Tell me more about that?" then you have to unpack the objection. You have to know the reason and then you fire the next gun.

Patient: No, I don't see what you see
You: Why?, What makes you say that?
Patient: Well, because of this, this,
You: You see, the real beauty of the treatment is

and then you fire the next gun, that you had saved up from the presentation. You did not fire that gun in the presentation.

You should anticipate the objections, adding positives, and removing negatives. There are a lot of objections that come over and over again, like the price the most mentioned one. Or I have to talk with my wife about that and so on.

You have to anticipate this and know what to say when they come up.

The patient is always doing a mental calculation. His negative things to buy, his beliefs, and objections against your positive reasons to buy. It is like a mental scale and he has a lot of kilograms, or pounds, on one side (his beliefs and objections) and you put in positive things, reasons to buy, on the other side. And then your side becomes heavier.

Then you remove objections and misbeliefs of the patient from his side, and his side is becoming lighter. Then you add new things on your side, and all of a sudden the scale turns towards buying, he is always making this mental calculation.

You have to find out his beliefs, his objections, and take them out and put positive reasons on top of it. You knock reasons down, that is why you don't shoot all your guns in the presentation. You knock the reasons down with some guns that you still have, and suddenly one of them will be decisive. It puts the weight on the buying side.

The beauty is, you never know which one it will be. Will it be an emotional reason? Will it be a logical reason? You don't know.

If the patient is still not convinced, go to step number nine.

Step 9 – Looping Pattern

You go back. You loop, you need to raise the level of certainty. The idea is to raise the level of certainty of the patient, he should be certain about
- you,
- your treatment,
- your team or your office.

Maybe he is not yet convinced of one of these three things. You have to find out what it is, and you have to cater to that.

Present again in a different way and ask for the order again. He comes up with another objection, you loop back, you go back again, and present again, to cater to that objection, he just came up with.

You get the new objection, you start the loop again, and so on.

Looping means going back in this closing sequence to the presentation, in order to raise more the certainty in you, in your treatment and your team or your dental office.

Step 10 – Lower the Action Threshold

Step number 10, lower the action threshold. Everybody has a threshold before he starts an action. For a lot of people, it is very high. And for some people, it is very low.

Everybody needs a certain level of certainty. The more the certainty goes up, the more it goes towards the threshold where he makes the buying decision.

You can either raise the certainty or move down the action threshold so that he will decide to buy earlier, although his certainty is not as high as it should be for the normal state of his threshold.

They need a certain level of certainty, to be comfortable to say yes. It is different in everybody.
Use trigger words for that (see also chapter 25). These words, lower the action threshold unconsciously.

Step 11 – Raise the Pain Threshold

And you can also raise the pain threshold. If they are reminded what they don't like. If they are reminded what they want to run away from, maybe it's one tooth that is, so way outside the arch or so dark or so ugly or so small or so big. One thing or two things. If you then remind the patient the whole time about that, he feels his pain threshold.

If you push it up, then he doesn't need so much certainty before he makes the buying decision. They feel the need more and they lower their action threshold. By raising the pain threshold, the patient lowers for himself the action threshold.

Step 12 – Make Patients for Life

After you have closed, the most important thing is, that with the close the sale is not over. All the service you give when you make the treatment is very important.

And how you follow up, how you make the controls how you make the maintenance. This is so important in order to make patients for life. They have to experience, that your customer service is very important.

Your post-treatment follow-up and control convert them into raving fans and referrers.

And here the sales process again or the closing sequence.

AIM – Create Certainty

01 – Immediate Control
02 – Gather Information
03 – Build Rapport
04 – Transition
05 – Presentation
06 – Wrap-up your Recommendation
07 – Ask for the Order
08 – First Objection
09 – Looping Pattern
10 – Lower the Action Threshold
11 – Raise the Pain Threshold
12 Make Patients for Life

The aim is to create certainty.

First step: take immediate control, be perceived as an expert, be likable, small talk.

Second step: gather information. You have to see whether or not the patient is qualified. Does he have the needs, what pain points are there, and if he can afford the treatment.

Third step: build rapport. Tonality, body language, very important.

Fourth step: make the transition "based on what you have said to me, this is the best solution for you. Let me tell you why", and transition towards your presentation.

Fifth step: the real presentation. And don't fire all your guns in the presentation.

Sixth step: wrap up your recommendation. Raise the value.

Seventh step: ask for the order, close.

Eighth step: the first objection.

Ninth step: loop back. Make again the presentation, wrap up your recommendation, ask for the order. Second objection, loop back, make the presentation, fire the next gun, and so on. "The real beauty of the treatment is ….."

Tenth step: lower the action threshold

Eleventh step: raise the pain threshold

Twelfth step: make patients for life.

13
THE 5 STEPS OF THE COMMUNICATION PROCESS

In this chapter, we want to talk about the five steps of the communication process. You will learn what to do before the actual presentation. And what the patient has to know for sure during the presentation so that he understands completely what you say and owns that in his mind, and he's willing to say yes.

Pre-thoughts

The number one number mistake we make when presenting a treatment is, we present a treatment plan before the patient really owns the consequences of our diagnosis. With that, I mean, imagine you have diagnosed decay in one of the teeth. So the consequences would be the decay will get bigger and bigger and will eventually get to the pulp or a cusp will break down and he will need an inlay or onlay or a crown even, instead of a filling. Or he will need root canal treatment instead of just a filling. Those are the possible consequences of your diagnosis. He has to understand that *before* you offer your treatment option.

In dental school we have been trained to identify the problem, find the problem, and then present a solution but this omits the patient from the process. Of course, *we* know what the consequences are. Of course, *we* understand completely the consequences of what we have seen in the X-ray, in the mouth, in the pictures, but the patient doesn't understand. The patient is not a dentist.

In this process of presenting, we have to include the patient. If we include the patient, he is more willing to say yes to our different options because he understands. You should usually talk to the patients about the consequences first, not their treatment. That's what you should do. How?

Through a three-stage process, you present, explain, and then verify. These three stages are step number three in the five steps of the communication process.

Step 1 – New patient scheduling system

Step number one a new patient scheduling system that converts nine out of 10 calls into patients that really sit down in your chair.

It starts with good communication at the front desk. This high level of communication brings in more patients, converts more patients from the calls that come in. You have to train your front office and you have to train them in patient experience not only on the phone, but also on once the patient is in. This is a whole other book about patient experience and patient service and front office desk management.

Be aware, that the whole communication process starts with excellent communication at the front desk. But this is a book about patient communication and presentation skills of the doctor.

Step 2 – Pre-exam talk

Somebody has to talk to the patient before we do the actual exam. We need to find out what is going on with them before they see the doctor. Usually this should be done by the front desk staff or by the treatment coordinator, it depends on the structure of your office.

The purpose of this pre-exam talk is, first of all, it introduces the treatment coordinator or the front desk to the patient. They get to know your team, step by step. They get to build rapport and they don't talk about money the first time they meet. They will talk about money later. When you have presented the case, they have accepted it and they should pay for it. If we don't have to step number two, the step of the pre-exam talk, then the money talk would be the first contact from the patient with that front desk person and that's not a good starting point.

It is much better if they come in and they are greeted warmly and happily, and then we do this talk.

The second purpose of this talk is that it gives the doctor information about the state of mind of that patient towards getting ideal dentistry. How is the patient set in his mind towards getting ideal dentistry? We have to find out, and whether there are any obstacles towards getting ideal dentistry like time, finances, or fear. We have to find that out before the patient meets the doctor.

You can set the expectations for the appointment for the patient and make sure their expectations are met. You have to find also out what they expect from this appointment.

It uncovers also the patient's attitude, willingness, and purchasing power. We have to find all these things out, inside of this step number two, the pre-exam talk.

When you later go through your case presentation with the patient, you, as a doctor or as a hygienist, will match their needs and wants perfectly because you are informed beforehand what their needs and what their wants are. They will feel very understood and this is when trust begins to be established, the patient experience becomes much more positive.

And this goes a long way in the differentiation of you from all the other offices that are around you.

How does the pre-exam talk look like?

The patient comes in and the front desk sits down with that patient in the reception area, and says

"Hi, my name is Laura, and I'm the front desk manager or I am the treatment coordinator.

I usually meet with every new patient to make sure your expectations for today are met".

Then she waits for an acknowledgment.

"I will start by asking you a few questions" and then she starts a little bit of small talking about where they work, what they do, where they live, where they come from, the address, and they write down all these data. A little bit of small-talk is in there, and it's like 2 to 4 minutes, then the actual questions come.

The question number one would be

"what specifically made you call our office for an appointment?". You understand why they called us. Then

"what are your expectations for today's appointment?" and number three,

"have you ever had a negative experience in the dental office?". You find out about past experiences. And number four, "what would you improve in the appearance or health of your teeth?". You find out, what he is conscious of.

"And why?". What is their Why? Why would they do that? It is very important for you to present your treatment option, meeting exactly this "why".

"Let's say you have issues in your mouth. Do you prefer to save the teeth? Or to have them removed?". You might say what kind of question is that? It's obvious that they would prefer to save their teeth. It's not obvious. Not everybody is so keen on keeping their teeth or saving their teeth. You have to find out what is the attitude of that patient towards saving the teeth or let them be removed. Some people, and I don't understand that attitude, just want the teeth to be removed if there is any problem.

Of course, you have to decide whether or not you would remove them ethically with your conscience completely free. If not, you just send them to another dentist. You don't do that. But you need to know if they are willing to save the teeth and do whatever you need to do to save the teeth, or if they want to have them removed.

Next question:

"Is there anything that would stand in your way of getting the dentistry you need, like fear, time, finances?". Let them answer that question.

"Do you have any questions for me?".

Through this question that the front office manager or the treatment coordinator responds, you also find out expectations.

Then the front desk manager or the treatment coordinator resumes
- what he or she has found
- what they came in for today.
- asks if they have additional problems like pain or sensitivity.
- they tell the patient that they will go over this with the doctor and that he or she will probably touch base on a few things.

Then the treatment coordinator or the front desk manager introduces their dental assistant.

Step 3 – 3 Stages Presentation

Before that

This is the actual presentation. And before you do the actual presentation, you go through

- the patient's health history,
- the pre-exam talk annotations, so what your treatment coordinator or your front desk manager found out and wrote down. You just go through that very quickly.
- and your diagnostics, x rays pictures, exam.

If you have not made anything of the last point, then you do the exam, you do the X rays, you do the pictures, and then you go through that before you start the presentation to the patient.

The 3 Steps

Now you know what the patient needs, wants, and is expecting. You are well prepared for your presentation. Then you do the presentation in three steps. You present, explain and verify. This idea is based on a system that is called "problem agitate solution" developed for writing advertising copy. You find a problem, you agitate the problem, you bring it to the surface, you make them feel the pain, pain in the mind, not in the mouth, and then you present a solution.

You need to sell them based on emotional reasons. Most patients are not going to buy your dentistry because it's *the right thing to do*. The only problems we are interested in solving are the ones we have an emotional connection to. Health is a very personal matter, there is an emotional connection to health.

Make them aware of the problems through agitation. This agitation is uncomfortable for the patient. Most dentists are used to avoid agitation, they want to avoid uncomfortable situations for the patient.

But if the patient is not uncomfortable with the situation he is in, he does not want to change that situation. And your treatment presentation has exactly the outcome or the aim to make the patient change his situation.

You need to make him understand and agree with the adverse consequences. Only then they will be willing to listen to your solution.

The three-stage presentation
present, explain, verify

Present: you show the diagnosed condition with objective instruments, photos, x-rays, then you
Explain: you talk about the consequences of non-treatment, that is your explanation and that is the most important part of this presentation and then you
Verify: that they see the diagnosis as seriously as you see it. In case, the patient does not say, I want to know how to fix that. He understands it and he wants to fix that.

If he does not say that, then you should verify. You should ask "how would you feel about that?", or "what do you think about that?". Verify, did they understand it? Do they see it as seriously as you see that situation?

If they don't feel pain, it is not obvious to them. It might be obvious to you, but not to them.

Find out and differentiate, what is the patient aware of and what shows up in the X-ray or exam. A lot of times it is very different, what they are aware of and what shows in the X-ray or the exam.

You need to put the level of awareness exactly where you are by showing them what happens if they don't make anything.

You need them to tell *you* that they don't like that. They don't like the situation they will be in, if you would not do anything. And they want to know how to fix it. You need them to say that.

They should tell you: that's not a good situation, what can we do about it? The patient will give you the reason why he wants the problem to be solved. And now he's engaged in the solution. This way, he is very interested in getting to know the possibilities of the solution to that problem. And you present these possibilities.

You need to transfer the ownership of the problem from you to him. What do I mean with ownership from you? Well, you own the problem at that moment. Why? Because you have diagnosed that problem, you know the problem and you are concerned about *his* problem. You own his problem at that moment. Now you need to get the ownership of that problem to him. If he is not aware, he doesn't care.

It is not giving him any pain. He doesn't own the problem. He has the problem but he doesn't own the problem (in his mind). He has to see it as *his* problem (which it is of course) to increase case acceptance and appointment show-up rate.

The patient has to fully understand, what you know is going on in his mouth.

Step 4 - Close

After that, you have to close. Closing is part of another book I wrote about "Sales Skills".

But you have to comfortably present the fee, close and gain financial commitment. You can do that in two ways.

- By committing the patient to pre-pay a certain amount. In this case, he has a financial commitment or
- by signing an informed consent that includes a financial agreement.

Step 5 – Track and improve your Funnel Statistics

See also chapter 6 in this book, to remember the sales funnel. It is very important to track your funnel statistics. The conversion of calls that come into the front office to new patients, and conversion of new patients to patients who have said yes, who have paid, and to whom you have made the treatment.

If you know these numbers, you know where you will have to improve your communication skills and your communication process.

THE PRESENTATION

14
BASIC THOUGHTS ON TREATMENT PRESENTATIONS

In this chapter, we want to talk about basic thoughts on treatment presentations. You will learn the different prerequisites for a successful presentation and what you have to be aware of and train for a successful presentation.

Patients are not educated in dentistry

You have to know patients are not educated in dentistry. You need to make sure your patients understand what is likely to happen to their teeth and their mouth without the treatment you recommend.

They have to see the consequences. You will have to explain that in a way they understand, not in dental talk. The best way is to show them pictures. This is happening to other patients that have the same problem and did not do anything about it. These are the consequences, show them.

Break it down

Then break it down into digestible chunks for the patient and make it easy for them to buy. If you overwhelm the patient with a complex treatment plan that is going to cost thousands of dollars, what do they do? They switch off their mind and as they are not in any immediate pain, they are likely to put another lifestyle purchase in priority and not the dental treatment.

Provide several options for payment

In reality, it's not about how much it costs. It's about how you pay for it. I repeat that again. The important thing is not how much it costs. The important thing is how you pay for it.

How much it costs you per month? How do you pay for it, you get it now and you pay for it later.

For example, you can make a 5% discount for full payment in advance. Accept all major credit cards. For larger cases, half up-front and the other half before the completion of the treatment, or third party or outside patient financing.

All the things are a possibility to make it easy for the patient to say okay, that's convenient for me. I will do it. You have to provide several options for payment.

Be persistent

We cannot tell the patient only one time what he needs and expect and rely on him to follow through on it, always. That's not going to happen.

You have to be persistent in your explanation. You have to repeat that over and over again during your presentation. They have to be fully convinced of the importance and feel psychologically ready to act on it.

Create a calm atmosphere.

If you need to do it in the operatory room, if you don't have a meeting room or something similar, and you need to do it in the operatory room, then sit the patient up, knee to knee, eye to eye level, not to make it threatening for him.

The patient should not be receiving information in an environment that is threatening to him.

Use visual aids

People remember 90% of what they see, and only 10% of what they hear. That's why intraoral cameras, imaging systems, digital x-rays are great educational tools. Even your cell phone, take pictures with it, and show them to the patient.

This helps the patient to feel that he or she is an active participant in the process. And it empowers the patient to make his or her own decision.

You go through these visual aids with them, together with them, explain to them what you see, so that they see the same thing.

Be enthusiastic.

You add value to their lives. You are helping your patients get good feelings about what they buy and mostly about themselves. That's what you do. So be enthusiastic about it.

You need to ask your patient, what is important to them and then you provide it to them.

"If there were anything we could change about your smile, what would it be?" Then he tells you what he would change. You change that. That makes him happy. You are making people happy, be enthusiastic about it.

And this enthusiasm is contagious. The patient is not buying just the service and what it can do. He is not buying just a treatment and what the treatment does. He is buying how it will make him feel. This is what he is buying.

Your patients don't buy the hard, cold facts on the treatment. They buy the warm people benefits.

Make it fun

Make it fun for them. Put yourself in the place of the patient. When you feel that you are being sold, you question the intent of the other person. The opposite happens when you are buying.

Buying is fun, being sold is not fun.

You understand the difference. Buying is active, being sold is passive. It is fun, you enjoy buying.

Usually, in order to know how to sell something effectively, remember how you enjoy buying when you bought something, a car or a big television or a vacation. When you bought that, how good you felt. Remember that and try to duplicate that feeling in the patient, when they buy your dentistry, your treatments. Help your patient to see the value of the service and start enjoying the good feelings they want.

Visualize the happy ending for the patient and the closing of the sale. Your goal is to help your patients see their own happy ending. Because buying is always more fun than being sold it generates excitement. You're helping them to want what they need. If they want it, and they buy it. They are happy about it.

If they don't want it and they just need it, and in the end, they buy it (because they need it, but they don't want it), they have been sold.

Positive Body Language

Have a positive body language, your body speaks volumes. Use open gestures, positive facial expressions.

Show interest in what the patient is telling you. Really pay attention. Show him with your face and with your attitude that you are paying attention by actively listening.

Listen to their thoughts. Don't do all the talking, but do (nearly) all the listening.

There are two golden rules for case presentations.

First rule: the more the dentist talks, the lower the case acceptance.

Second Rule: the more the patient talks, the higher the case acceptance.

In the end, there is only one rule.
Don't talk too much!

Positive thinking attracts positive results

Before the presentation, say to yourself: "I see the advantages of my services, of my treatments. I see the advantages when I touch the patient's mouth, this is going to be really good for the patient. And I see the happy ending."

Consciously choose to use positive thoughts because they will guide your unconscious mind. Your mind and you are going to guide the mind of the patient.

See the advantages of the treatments. Combine this with how to solve the problem of the patient. Visualize the happy ending, seeing the other person using and benefiting from what he or she buys: veneers, smile makeover, or an orthodontic treatment.

You should be feeling good about it, you have to visualize it and then you feel happy about it and you transmit this enthusiasm and this happiness to the patient. Make them feel good during the presentation.

Make them feel good

Help people get good feelings about the treatment and about themselves. Remember, people buy based on emotions and feelings. They don't buy based on hard facts and cold facts. Make your patients get good feelings about the treatment and about themselves. If they feel good, they like you. If they feel good about the treatment, they want the treatment.

Ask

Discover your patient's needs simply by asking. Ask "have" and "want" questions. Help your patients to recognize what they really want.

- What do you like most about what you already have?
- What do you like most about your smile right now?

Then you know what you don't have to change. Followed by

- What don't you have that you want?
- What would you like to have in your smile and you don't have that?

Then you know what you have to change. Or:

- Would it be fair to ask what you like least about what you've got?

Listen and resume

Actively listen to the patient and acknowledge his concern.

Summarize and then paraphrase, to show that you understand. You take the words of the patient, you change these words, you just repeat what they said.

Tie problems and solutions together.

"Based on what you've told me (problem) about your smile. I'd like to suggest this treatment solution".

What a patient really wants is to know is: "what's in it for me?". You have to tell him what's in it for him.

The risk of No and the benefit of Yes

Discuss the risk and consequences of not having the treatment. Discuss the benefits of the treatment.
-   You will have a better function.
-   Your excellent health will be restored.

Incentives for the patient

Sometimes patients need incentives to move forward. Give them an incentive.
-   You will look better.
-   You will feel better.
-   You will taste your food better.
-   Your smile will be gorgeous.

In this stage is where the patient will decide based on the incentives.

Summarizing the presentation process

If the patient trusts you, feels the need of doing something about his problems, knows that you can help him to get the good feeling he wants.

What could possibly prevent him from taking action?

Well, that's a good question. And this is exactly what you may have to ask.

What could possibly prevent you from taking action right now?

What is preventing you from taking action right now?

When you ask for the close, and they say, let me think about it. Then you have to say: if everything is clear, what prevents you from taking action?

You have to understand the objection. Objections are discussed in other chapters.

15
POWERFUL QUESTIONS DURING THE PRESENTATION

In this chapter, we will talk about the powerful questions during the presentation. You will learn the goals of asking, and the different questions you should ask.

Goals when asking

The goal of asking questions is to identify the patient's "why". Their reason
- why they want to change,
- why they want an improvement,
- why they want the teeth to be fixed.

You might detect some misalignment or you might detect some uncommon color and sizes of the teeth. But maybe it's not *their* reason to want to change, to have an improvement.

You need to understand why *they* want to change and then cater to that reason. You have to show that your treatment exactly serves for that reason. It will solve the problem of that "why". Not any other problem. Then it is the right thing for the patient to do. So that's the idea of asking questions, it is to identify the patient's why.

You have to memorize the questions that I will give you during this chapter. Pick out some of the questions and memorize them so that they come easily when you ask them.

General Questions

In general, you should have a nice body language. The body language is always important. You have to lean forward a little bit. Make eye contact and smile. You have to signal with your body language that you are here to help and that you have the best interest of the patient in mind.

That's what you want to achieve with your body language. Without saying it, you show it.

Avoid yes or no questions also. You need to make questions to the patient, so that he starts talking and explaining, that's how you can gather information for yourself. And that information is important for you to understand what he really wants.

Have your outcome in mind. What's your outcome? The acceptance of the treatment that you want to offer.

Your questions are aimed towards gathering information from the patient of what he wants. Then think, what would be the best treatment to achieve his wants, and then you explain to the patient the best treatment later, not now.

What motivated you to come here today?

One of the first questions you should ask is "what motivated you to come here today?" With that, you gather information and motives of the patient.

He talks, don't interrupt him. Why did he come? You write down, you take notes, and then you continue with follow-up questions. That means, you take the notes, and he stops talking and then you say:

"You said this or that. Can you explain that a little bit better?"

That's a follow-up question. Or

"can you specify that a little bit more?"

Just like this, or if he said: "I want to improve my smile"

"In what sense do you want to improve your smile?"

All these questions you make follow-up on what he said. The first question is always the most difficult one, and then all the others result from the answers to the first question and the consecutive questions.

Exactly what are we trying to accomplish here today?

That is a very outcome-driven question. We ask, what is he expecting? Very goal-oriented.

What is their goal? What do they want? Write that down. They will tell you what they want and what they need.

It's not like "how can I help you?". It's not the same question.

Big picture Questions

The following type of questions is the big picture questions. Later you go into detailed questions. In the big picture questions, you let the patient talk. Use the answers that he gives you, later in your sales pitch. That means when you start to do the closing, when you ask the patient to go ahead with the treatment to say yes, you will do the treatment, and let's start. That's a close. If you help the patient to make the close, you will use the answers to these big picture questions that he gave you.

You will take this information that you wrote down, and then say: exactly as you told me that you wanted this and that, this treatment accomplishes this and that. Then it is a no-brainer for him to accept the treatment later, but you need that information.

Otherwise, you don't know what exactly he is looking for. And maybe your treatment is really good, but it's not exactly what he is looking for.

What don't you like about your mouth?
….and how do you want it to be or look like?

What don't you like, of your mouth? And how do you want it to be or to look like?

Let him talk. A similar, but a softer question of this would be:

Where are you today? And where do you want to be with your smile or with your teeth?

And what would you change or improve in your smile?

What would you change or improve of your teeth?

What seems to be the problem?
….and how long have you had this problem?

This is another big picture. It aims at the pain point. Now we are talking about a problem. Not about what he likes or not. What's the problem? And how long have you had the problem? The patient starts to feel uncomfortable. That is what we want.

You start to search in his mind, his frustrations. You start to provoke emotions in his mind. And this is very important because he will only accept your treatment if the treatment really solves his problem. And for this purpose, he first has to be aware of his problem. So, you ask directly about the problem. That's one of the possible questions. No pain, no sale. Not pain in the mouth, pain in the mind.

A similar question would be:
What is your biggest headache with your teeth?
What is your biggest headache with your smile?

If this consultation accomplished everything you could possibly hope for, what would that look like?

This is another big picture question. Here we paint a picture in the patient's mind of what would be the ideal situation he is looking for.
A similar question could be:

How would this consultation be a success for you?

The patient says X,
and then you say: what else would make it a success?
Patient: Y
You: what else?
Patient: Z
You: what else?

Then you know what he's looking for. You can ask many times "what else". And you write down everything. This is what he wants. That is very important information for you.

A lot of dentists assume they know what the patients want. It's not like that. A lot of patients really don't want what the dentist thinks of. They have to be asked.

A lot of dentists assume they know how they have to treat the patient. But some patients are different. Some patients need extra things to make an appointment, a consultation successful. You don't know, what the patient is looking for. Why don't you ask?
That is why these questions are important.

What is your ultimate objective?

Another big picture question could be what is your ultimate objective? That is how you understand the goals and objectives of the patient.

What would be your ideal situation?

This is another big picture question. Ask to be as specific as possible
"Please be very specific in what is ideal for you"

Specific Questions

Then there are specific questions. They are aimed to find out the pain. Again, not the physical, but the mental pain.

Of all the factors that you mentioned, what is the most important one for you?

What is he ultimately trying to accomplish? That what's really the factor?
In the end, you don't need 100 reasons to sell a treatment. The patient does not need 100 reasons to buy a treatment. He only needs one. And what's the most important thing for him to cater to? This *one* reason!

Have I asked about every detail that is important to you?

That's a very important question. Anything we have missed? Then the patient can think again of everything. And maybe he says, Is there any pain involved? For example. Then you answer: that's the good part of it. Bla bla bla. "That's the good part of it" one of the closing techniques in my "Sales Skills" book.

You answer any concerns he might have with: that's the best

part of it. That's a good part of it. And then you answer to that objection or question. So, the patient can think of what is also important to him and we have not discussed or he has not talked about.

Any additional concerns?

What do we want to achieve? Slowly, the patient should feel uneasy. He feels the problem bigger than initially. That's the important thing by asking questions about the problems. We put the problems now first in his mind. And they start to be bigger for him. That's good for us because then we can offer him a solution he's interested in.

We have to increase his pain in the mind.

Ways not to fire all your guns

You should not fire all the guns. You need some guns for the objections part.

- Do not narrate the patient's answer. You don't ask something he answers and then you say "I know that this is like this" No, let him talk. And then at the end with your treatment presentation, narrate the patient's answer not now.
- Do not comment.
- Feel the patient's pain, feel when he really is upset or when he really feels. He's talking about something that bothers him, a problem. If you feel that you might notice what is important of what he said.
- Let him know you understand his specific problems. Let him know you care about his answers.
- Let him know you will do everything you can to help him reach his goal.
- And listen, don't talk, let him talk.

Invasive Questions

These questions are aimed to qualify the patient.

Qualifying means, whether or not the patient needs, wants, can pay, and feels an urgency to have the treatment done.

You have all your information and now you need to know whether or not the treatment you will offer is the right one for him, and if he can pay it.

How long have you been thinking about that?

You find out if there is any urgency now. Similar question:
How long have you been wanting to
- get new teeth,
- get a fixed prosthesis,
- get your teeth fixed,
- get a beautiful smile?

How much have you been thinking of investing in this treatment?

This is a money question. Here the use of tonality is very important. Show him that it's important to invest in health and you are expecting an investment.

Find out whether or not your treatment is the correct one for him and if he can afford it.

Only move forward if both criteria are fulfilled.

16
3-STEP TECHNIQUE FOR PATIENTS TO SAY YES

In this chapter, we will talk about a three-step technique for patients to say yes to your treatments. Learn the three steps and how to apply them to dentistry.

Change

If you want people to do something, you want them to change. Change their current situation, change their opinion, and nobody wants to change because they are comfortable. It is difficult to get patients to say yes.

Step 1 – Want

The first step is called "want".
Ask a plan-based question. What do they want, concerning their future, and then they open up.
- what smile
- what gum
- what teeth do they want to have in the future?

All this, based on the pain points they have now. Chances are their comments are positive it puts them into a positive mindset.

So, in the future I would like to have a bright smile and smile at the wedding of my daughter or something like that.

Step 2 - Feel

The second step would be "feel".

People make decisions based on emotions and later justify them with logic. They decide upon what feels right, not on what makes sense or what should be done, or what is the correct thing to do. If it feels right, they do it.

You need to evoke feelings in them. The second step is to provoke feelings. Like the feeling about the situation and the future.

If you ask people to describe an emotion, they get (feel) a bit of that emotion at that moment. With a question about how they would feel in the future, you put them in a good place thinking about their happy point in the future.

Step 3 - Uncomfortable

Step three, make him uncomfortable. Remove the comfort they are in right now.

People don't move to get more comfort now. But they move when they are uncomfortable now.

You need to make him aware that he's not comfortable right now.

What are the consequences if we do nothing? That's very important, that makes his comfort go away. Because the dream he described in step one will not become a reality. And on top of that, you can make him see that his situation right now, where there is a problem, will get worse with time.

These two things,
- his dream will not become true and
- his situation will get worse.

They want to get away from that double-bad situation.

The three steps are
1 ask a plan based question about the future,

2 how are they going to feel when they get there, of course good.
- What will you do?
- What will you do with your implant fixed prosthesis?
- What are you going to eat?
- Where will you smile?
- Think of all these pictures where you will have a beautiful smile.
- What about your granddaughter? When she loves your smile,
you put the patient at a feeling level. Positive feelings. Let them describe that.

3 then let them describe the situation, what happens if it doesn't work out?

You have to make them see two things. The dream is not going to happen. And second, it's going to get worse than it is now.

That doesn't mean they will buy, that it means they are in a position now where they are prepared to accept the change.

Remember, it's very difficult to make people change. They don't want to change because they're comfortable right now. And they don't want to change to be more comfortable in the future. The only want to change if they are uncomfortable right now.

Present a solution to fix their problem. That's your presentation.

And by saying: Good news, you are in the right place, we can help you! Then how you are going to help him, based on what he said.

17
OVERCOMING BARRIERS DURING THE PRESENTATION

In this chapter, we want to talk about how to overcome barriers. You will learn what the possible barriers could be and how to overcome them. And what to avoid during the presentation.

The Process

Now that you know what to do before, during, and after the presentation, here are some guidelines to help you through the process.

First of all, you have to set the agenda, then state the value and co-discover with the patient the value. Then you check for the agreement, and then you move to the close.

That's how you move forward.

For example, you set the agenda by saying

"What I want to discuss with you today is how we can fix your smile". Then, you co-discover the value with a patient:

"So, then we can decide what's best for your health and best for your beauty".

"How does that sound?", here you check for agreement.

"There are four phases to your treatment plan. This is what we are going to do first", then you start to close with the patient.

Use a confident delivery throughout the presentation. You have to sound confident. You have to be convinced by your own offer. If you're not convinced you cannot convince anybody.

And make positive assumptions. Think the patient will go forward with the treatment.

Start off strong in your presentation. People usually remember the first and the last things you say and they forget everything in the middle.

So, use a closure statement for the finale. "Here is how we are going to help you..."

Barriers for the Patient

What barriers could be there? The primary reason for patient hesitation is, that
-   they are not convinced of the need,
-   they are afraid or
-   they cannot pay (they have money worries).

All three things lead to the patient saying no to your treatment offer and they don't make an appointment to move forward.

Not convinced of the need

You have not created urgency and value in the treatment. The consequences of delaying the treatment have not been explained well enough. The pain inside of the mind of the patient has not been increased and there is no understanding. He does not see what you see in his mouth. You have not explained the status and what will happen if we do nothing.

The patient is not clear about the severity of the problem. The patient believes that if it doesn't hurt me, I can wait until it does. A lot of patients think that and you have to take them out of that belief and into a belief of: if I do nothing, it gets worse and it will be much more expensive to fix that.

Fear

You should invest in comfort options for your patients. Get to the cause of the patient's fear and address it. And you have to tell the patient that you can remove that cause by having amenities blankets, pillows, and anesthesia, nitrous oxide, sedation dentistry, all these things are important to have in your office for fearful patients.

Fearful patients, they might already know what they need. They might be convinced that it is necessary and urgent. They might have the money to pay it, but they don't make the next step because they fear the situation.

They fear that it will do some harm to them or similar things. Fear can be many different things. It can be:
- this is going to hurt or
- it will fall out immediately.

Different patients fear different things. You might assume that they fear pain, but maybe they don't fear pain.
- They fear it's going to take too long.
- They fear that it will not hold in their mouth.
- They fear that it will fall out.
- They fear that they will have sensitivity afterward.

If you don't ask about the fear they have, you will not find out what they fear. And if you don't find out what they fear, you cannot address it. Find out the fear they have. It's not always pain.

Money

The number three is money worries. Let patients know that you have different options for payment, have multiple third-party financing options available for your patients.

Let them know that you are flexible. But make sure the patient is clear on your parameters.

Role of the Front Desk

The role of the front desk is very important. Your front desk coordinator is the last person your patient sees before leaving the office.

He or she must be well trained to be a closer. I know *you* have to close. But if you close and the patient is still not completely convinced, then the front desk has to go ahead and close (again).

The front desk has to be ready for additional questions from the patient. They have to be trained on that, and has to have great verbal skills, about finances as well as dental procedures.

They also have to be able to read the body language of hesitant patients and pinpoint the concerns. Get them out of the way these concerns. Clarify everything. Make it clear.

Imagine the patient has been closed, but while the patient is paying, the front desk notices something is not completely correct. Then they should ask!

"How can I help you to be very clear about the procedure?" "Well, I have not understood the doctor completely about this and that", so the front desk explains the rest.

What to avoid

You should not rush through the presentation.

You should not assume that the patient has fear or has no money. Many patients you think they have no money, find a way to pay your treatments because they are convinced and they want it.

Talking too much and talking about yourself. And listening too little. You should listen much more than you talk.

You should not include unnecessary details in your presentation. That makes everything very confusing, overloaded, overwhelming for the patient.

You should not release patients too soon for the financial discussion. If the patient is not ready, he cannot be put into the financial discussion. He has to be convinced. He has to want the treatment completely.

And he has to be clear about the options that he has and about the procedure itself.

18
MISTAKES DURING THE CASE PRESENTATION

In this chapter, we want to talk about the mistakes you can do during the case presentation. You will learn the possible mistakes, how to avoid them, and how to use them for you.

You will see that at the end of the day, the case presentation is less about the treatment itself. And it's much more about the patient and understanding the patient. I think in the last chapters, you have understood that and one of the most important things is your body language.

Mistake 1: Body Language not OK

Your body language should be congruent. Your facial expressions should really show
- that you are interested,
- that you are excited about the treatment,
- that you are happy
- that you are enthusiastic.

If your facial expression is like a poker face or you even shows a bad mood, that would be a disadvantage. Nobody wants to be with a bad-mooded dentist.

Lean forward towards the patient. Maintain eye contact at eye level with the patient. Do not be over the level of the patient, but on the same level as the patient.

Mistake 2: Talking too much about the features

A feature is what the treatment does.
A benefit is what the treatment does for the patient.

Have you noticed the difference?
You have to talk about the benefits, not the features.

An example of a feature: cleaning the teeth from stone.
What it does for the patient: it makes his teeth and his gums healthier so that they stop bleeding. That's a benefit, not a feature.

You concentrate on the benefits, not on the features. Usually dentists talk too much about the features.

Patients always need to know what's in it for them.
You need to tell them: "here is exactly what it means for you".

For example, you explain a feature.
"I put an implant into the bone". But ask yourself, what does it do for the patient?
"With an implant, I can fix your teeth in your mouth. And this makes it possible that you bite on an apple just like that, without your teeth falling out or your teeth moving. Really with confidence. You can eat again!", that's a benefit. It's not a feature.

Mistake 3: Concentrating on educating the patient

Patient education only will not make them accept your proposal. Understanding the patient is the driver, connect with the patient and then he has the impression of being understood.
This is much more important for the patient in order to say

yes, than to be educated on how an implant works.

"First, we do the surgery, we make a hole in your bone, and put an implant in". They don't want to hear that.

They want to hear what's in it for them and they want to know that you care about their needs, their wishes, their wants.

If they know that you care, then they are ready to say yes to your treatment. That builds confidence.

Mistake 4: Not having enough time

Don't start a presentation if you don't have enough time, don't start it at all. You will not be able to find out what you need, build rapport, increase the pain, explain your solution, and ask the patient to accept your treatment.

For all this, you need time. If you don't have enough time, schedule a new appointment. If you are too busy, then schedule it right before or after your office hours. In most of the cases 20 minutes to half an hour will do.

Mistake 5: No time to get to know the patient

This is an important one, small-talk is essential and very important. The small-talk you do before you even take a mirror and look into the patient's mouth. That is where a lot of the basis is constructed for confidence and trust.

Patients want you to get to know them better. Also related to the treatment, you can ask things not only of their life but also related to their smile, their past experiences with the dentist, and so on.

They want you to know:
- why THEY want the treatment and
- how it must fit into their lives.

They need confidence in you. Not why *you* would do the treatment, know why *they* want the treatment. And also how it must fit into their lives. That would be their lifestyle. Do they have enough time? Can they come in during the week or do you have to open a Saturday for them?

How do you get the confidence of the patient? Confidence builder could be

-   thoroughness during the exam, you use loops or a microscope. Also, in your hygiene appointment, which would be the first clinical contact of your patient with your office (except in emergencies), if your hygiene appointment follows a strict protocol and the protocol is explained step by step while the hygienist is doing the procedure to the patient. They have the impression that you follow other protocols than others. You don't, but you explain to the patient what you're doing at that moment. And you're the only office who does that. So, they assume you're doing something different, but you don't. And then because you do something different (in their minds) and you follow a strict protocol, they think you are really organized and very thorough in what you do. And that builds confidence.
-   The appearance of the office, the appearance of you and the staff builds confidence.
-   Efficiency and friendliness of you and your staff.
-   Having a conversation about his or her "why". Why the patient wants the treatment.
-   If you show you are curious about their circumstances, their lifestyle, their schedule, and how you can fit the treatment in, this also builds confidence for them. They gain certain confidence with the fact, that you are interested in really helping them because you try to adapt yourself to them, not them to your schedule. "Well, we are free on Friday, we can do that on Friday". But what about the patient?

Do you get it? It is very important to adapt to the patient. You have to adapt to the needs of the patient, and then you make it easy for them to say yes. This generates confidence.

Maybe they never had before a healthcare provider that asks this type of questions, that really was willing to address to their needs and their lifestyle. That builds confidence.

And all this you can do in less than 10 minutes. It is not something that you have to invest a lot of time. It is just five to ten minutes of your time and you have a patient for life that is convinced that you are the one and you are the best.

Mistake 6: Explaining the HOW too much

Another mistake could be explaining the how too much. They don't need to know exactly how you fix their teeth. How you put in the implant in the bone, how you prep for the veneers, how you cement the veneers. They don't need that.

They need to learn that you understand why they want to fix it. And that your treatment option caters to exactly that "why". And how it must fit into their lifestyle.

They assume you know how to fix it. You don't have to explain that (except if they ask) or show that you know a lot about dentistry. They assume that. That is why they are sitting in your chair.

The perfect statement

Dear patient, I understand that you are really looking forward to (the why). The why of the patient. For example. A woman wants to fix her smile because her daughter is going to marry. Why does she want to fix her smile? The first thing is because her daughter will marry and she wants to smile in the pictures. And she wants to be happy that day. Not because her teeth are crooked or something like that. No, because of the wedding. You have to find that out. In this case: "Dear patient I understand that you are really looking forward to your daughter's wedding and to smile at that wedding. Like you have never smiled before."

I know this is important for you. You mentioned the why and you say this is important for her and that you know that.

I am confident we can help you to get that done. What do you think the patient will think? You are the doctor, he or she will do the treatment with. Then then you state that you've done that many, many times.

We have helped many other patients in that situation.

You also told me that you are very busy during the week. Together with the treatment coordinator (or the front desk manager), *we will work out a perfect plan that fits into your schedule* (lifestyle).

That would be a very good sequence to get through that presentation.

Here again:

Dear patient, I understand that you are really looking forward to (the why).

I know this is important for you.

I am confident we can help you to get that done.

We have helped many other patients in that situation.

You also told me that you are very busy during the week.

Together with the treatment coordinator (or the front desk manager), we will work out a perfect plan that fits into your schedule (lifestyle).

The truth

The truth is that the case presentation influences patients by providing the experience of being understood.

It has nothing to do with your treatment plan. It has to do with the impression of the patient, that you understood him. And then they assume that the treatment plan that you give is exactly the one that they need. You are the expert.

You don't need to explain the features of the treatment. You have to make them see you understood completely what they need. If they have that feeling, the acceptance of the treatment is nearly for sure. Nearly 100% done.

Informed Consent conversations after the presentation fulfill your medical-legal obligations, so you don't have to explain the advantages, disadvantages, contraindications, indications, the treatment options during your presentation. If the patient asks for it, it's ok to provide that information. But the patient has to be convinced you understood what he needs.

Mistake 7: Questions you should not ask

1 What are you using now? And how is it going for you?

These questions are not bad, but don't ask two-part questions. Ask first one part, let him talk. And then the other part.

2 Any questions the patient might have already answered during the conversation. He will think you didn't listen to him. And it sounds robotic. Like if you were following a script. You can follow a script, you can write down questions that you always have to ask from the chapter about powerful questions. You might pick out some questions and ask these questions over and over again, with every patient, and then of course, you have a script. But if, before that question comes up, the patient in his statements has already answered that question, without you having made that question, you just don't have to bring up that question anymore, because it's already answered. It would show

that you don't listen and that you follow a script, and it's a quick way to lose your business.

Mistake 8: Not showing interest

Imagine the patient talks too long. Very long about how he loves soccer, for example, in the small-talk, because yesterday was a game and he loves soccer and in the small talk he's talking a lot about that. And then he asks you if you like soccer. And you say politely:

No, I don't like soccer. I like more tennis.

Why would you say that? Don't say that. Even if you hate soccer, don't say so. You say instead:
I would love to try it one day, or
I don't have enough time nowadays to dig deeper into it, but I would love to.

That's it. So, you make him understand you have no idea about soccer, but not because you hate it, but because you have no time. And soccer is only an example.

Remember

Remember, you need to be just like them.
Your body language and tonality show them that you are there to help the patient.

ADDITIONAL TIPS AND TRICKS

19
ACTIVE LISTENING

In this chapter, we want to talk about active listening and how to practice that with your patient. You will learn to let patients talk and how to send signals, you are still active and listening to them.

This is a very small chapter about how to reinforce the patient to talk and you just listen and take your notes and extract the data that you need.

Dentists talk too much. Usually they talk too much to the patient, the more the dentist talks, the lower the case acceptance, and the more the patient talks, the higher the case acceptance.

I have repeated that in many chapters.

<u>Listening</u>

Listening is an active act of trying to understand what someone is saying to you. You have to focus on the patient. While he speaks, don't think "What will I respond to that?". No, let him talk and focus on what he is saying.

Periodically restate what he says. You say:

To be sure I understand. It sounds like you're saying this and that.
Or
If I'm hearing you correctly, you're saying this and that.

This shows you are listening.
First, it shows you're listening.
And second, it gives him the chance to clarify if you misunderstood something.

From time to time restate what he says. Just repeat what he has just said in order to make sure you have understood correctly, and to give him the chance, if you misunderstood, to make it clear to you.

When you have a question.

Before you go on, let me make sure I understand.
And then you ask your question, or
A moment ago, you said this and that, can you give me clarification about that?

Then you have to show you are listening.
The body language is important.
Nod your head.
Maintain eye contact with the patient while he's speaking.
You say, huh, mm-hmm, Mm-hmm.
Or you say yes. Or okay.

Just to show that you are following him, and you understand and you are there, present, you are with him.

And take notes. Not with a computer, with paper and a pencil. Later you put that into the computer, but take notes. And this shows you are engaged, but not interrupting.

Try not to interrupt the patient while he is talking. This is very helpful for the patient so that he can explain everything that he thinks of. And after he stopped, you can make follow-up questions.

Let him talk more and more, and you can make questions that you want for your understanding to clarify things.

20
GIFT-WRAP YOUR VALUE

In this chapter, we want to talk about gift-wrapping your value.
You will learn the difference for your value if you wrap it and how to apply it to dentistry.

The best example to explain to you the gift wrapping of your treatment, increasing the value is the pen or watch example.

Imagine any pen or watch in any store. It's on the table or it's in a big box, together with 200 other pens or watches.
How much is the pen or the watch? You would say not very much.

Now take this pen or this watch and put it inside of a stand of Plexiglas. Only 12 pens or 12 watches are on the stand, and the manufacturer's name is on top of this Plexiglas stand and it's in a nice department store where you can buy it.
How much is the pen or watch now? Well, more. It has more value, the price is higher.

Now imagine this pen or watch in a wooden, high-quality box. And this box is inside of a big glass box with a spotlight on it. And it's in one of the finest shops in town. And to get to this watch or pen, you have to talk to the staff to open this glass box and the wooden box.

Now again, how much is the pen or watch? Much, much, more. Of course. So, what is the difference between these three examples?

It's everything that is *around* the thing that you are trying to sell. It's not only the treatment, that is worth the money. It is all the stuff that comes with it or is there around it.

You don't charge only for the treatment you charge for everything else, too.

The clearer you explain all of the things that are around your treatment, the easier it is for you to articulate the differences against or opposed to the similarities of your competitors.

The patient will compare your treatment always to the treatment of other competitors. But if

- your service is better,
- you are highly skilled to do the treatment because you've got a lot of continuing education,
- your staff is better trained,
- your customer service is exceptional,
- your guarantees are much higher,
- you use the best materials ever.

You have to communicate that.

Patients only see you are going to make a crown, and a competitor is also going to make a crown and then compare the two prices.

It is up to you to, first put some extra things on the treatment and second communicate them.

Make everybody know about your extra things that are around your treatments. Once everybody knows all these extras, they will not compare you anymore immediately to the other competitors.

They need to find out what the competitors have also on top

of the treatments. If these competitors don't communicate it, then they're supposed only to make the treatment and not something else around it.

Patients then will compare only the treatment of the competitors with your treatment plus all the benefits that you put on top of the treatment for your patient. Now the price difference is justified and the price difference is good.

It is easier for other people to find that value. Price and value are not the same. The price is the price that you come up with. The value is different for everybody.

For some people, it has a high value to have white teeth. For others, it's a low value, but the price is always the same. If I consider having white teeth very important. White teeth have a high value for me, the price is under my value. For me, the price looks cheap.

If for me it's not important to have whiter teeth, not at all, then for me this same price is too high.

In order to make people see that your value is higher than your price, you need to put the value in front of the eyes of the patient.

Let me give you an example. If one of your hands is the price, and the other one is the value. Imagine you are looking to a patient and you put the price-hand upfront towards that patient, exactly in the view of the patient, what appears bigger? Of course, the price-hand. The price appears bigger than the value, but if you put the value-hand in front of the price-hand, then all of a sudden, the price does not seem so high and so big and so important.

That is the idea of wrapping your value. Who hasn't bought something for more money than he said he would? Everybody! If you want to buy a car, you have a certain budget and in the end, you spend more. If you want to make a trip somewhere, you have something in mind and in the end, you spend more. It happens with nearly any service. In the end, you might spend more than you thought you would spend.

It is important to know that people don't have a budget in their mind. And second, it's important to know that all your treatments and all your prices are higher than what people thought they would cost.

Although your price is low, it still is higher than they thought it would cost. But people have desires and this is important. They are willing to pay for these desires.

What you have to do is to cater to these desires, how do you find them out? With your questions at the beginning of the sales process.

And then put your treatment with some added value that caters to the desires that the patient has. And push always this hot button of the desires the patient has.

People buy what they want, not what they need. So never overestimate the needs. You have to find out what they want.

Your job is to increase that desire. And put your value in front of the price. And then, after you showed the value, bring up the price with such killer confidence that you believe that it's worth it.

After you have built up the value after you have gift wrapped your treatment with the value and you have made it clear that it has a lot of value. Then you come up and say, it's only 1000 Euros.

"It's only 1000 Euros", with confidence in you, your team, and your treatment.

If **you** are not convinced, you cannot convince. So, if you don't believe in you, your treatment and your team, please don't expect somebody else to believe it.

First you have to be convinced. And if you are convinced, then it's contagious and the patient feels it.

So, how can you grift-wrap in dentistry? With your location first, if you want to open up a dental office, make it in one of the best regions of your town. Yes, you have to pay more in rent, and so on. But it's worth it to increase your prices and to have them at a high level. That is what high-level brands do in every city. They look for the best neighborhood or the best streets in town, and they put the shops there. They have to pay much more rent, but it's worth it because the margins are higher.

It's also how you act, how you dress, how you talk, how your office looks. So, it's worth it if you have already an office to redesign that office to make it look much better to make it worth your price.

Your staff, how well is it is trained, how it delivers customer service.

Your guarantees, your technology, your implant booklet. So If you use the most advanced technology people see that and then of course, that is an added value to your treatment.

Your implant booklet when you make the implants you just don't let the patient go. You give them a sort of implant passport.

You can do that same thing for crowns, veneers, even for fillings if you want. Like a guarantee card.

You can also make a like a booklet or a passport for your prophylaxis treatments. So the patient has an overview. Oh, I have been every year there or even twice a year. That is good. You put a stamp in and then it's nice. By the way the German Social Security System has that.

Then, how you present your veneers if they just come in, in a small device and they are inside of water, and you take them out, that has not a big value.

They should be in a nice frame and presented in a nice way. If your dental technician does not deliver them in a nice way, just put them yourself in a very nice presentation before the patient comes in. So he sees: Wow, that is a high quality, high value, piece of work.

You need to do that. If you don't do that, you cannot justify your price, if your prices are way higher than other competitors.

And also for example how your take-home kits for bleaching look like. If they look nice, if they have instructions in them that are beautiful and nicely done. If it is easy for the patient to handle. All of these things are very important.

For example, Invisalign™ has improved their take-home kits for the patient. It looks very high-end now.

21
SMALL TIPS AND TRICKS FOR CASE PRESENTATIONS

In this chapter, we want to talk about small tips and tricks for your case presentation, your treatment presentation. You will learn little things you have to be aware of, or change to make your presentation even more successful.

Planting a seed in the mind

Number one is planting a seed in the mind of the patient. How do you do that? What you can do is make the patient think in the direction you want him to think.

How do we let a kid know a story is coming? When you say: "Once upon a time", when you say that, children relax and think this is going to be good. And then they open their mind, they are now ready to get information and pictures and stories and think about what you are telling them. They open up, they relax and they are happy.

Of course, you cannot say "once upon a time" to a patient. But you can use the adult version of once upon a time to open the mind of the patient for your information, or to make him receptive to your information.

What is that adult version? The grown-up version is

"Just imagine"

Say 'just imagine', and then the patient's mind goes in the direction you will describe. By the way, you cannot NOT think about something that somebody tells you.

If I say to you: now don't think of an elephant what you see in your mind is an elephant, you cannot NOT think about an elephant. That is how this works.

So, you say, just imagine and then you open up the mind and you can plant the seed.

Just imagine what is it is going to feel like to have a gorgeous smile. The patient thinks about the feeling of a beautiful smile.

Just imagine what your husband will say, or your wife will say, when he or she sees you with that gorgeous smile.

You plant ideas in the head of the patient
- just imagine the feeling
- just imagine how confident you're going to feel when in the next business meeting you, before you make the close, show your really confident smile.

If you know that your patient is a businesswoman or a businessman. Just take some daily situations they live and now they should imagine these daily situations successfully, because of that new link that new smile, or with their new teeth, with their fixed teeth on implants.

- just imagine how confident you will be in the next family meeting. When you go to eat in a restaurant. That is a lot worth for these patients.

They cannot help but to see themselves in that scenario. And you have already gained a lot.

You use 'just imagine' to create visions for things patients really want. They want to run towards it.

But you can also use 'just imagine' to create visions of things they want to get away from.

You: Just imagine you are in a family meeting in a restaurant and your denture falls out.
Patient: Oh, I don't want that.
You: We can avoid that. Bla bla bla ...

You can increase pain also with "just imagine" and then you continue,

"wouldn't it make sense to do this or that today to get you to avoid this situation? "

That is a very good situation in the future that you opened his mind to see that right now.

Wouldn't that make sense?

Because indeed it makes sense. You have already directed the patient to want it.

Using the Schedule

Never start a presentation if there is no time to finish. If you need to reschedule, you say that you need more time for the patient and this amount of time that is left until the next patient comes is not enough.

Don't let them know what they need. Don't let them know

you will need three implants, don't say that. Don't give him a clue about what he needs and don't give him a clue about what it will cost.

If they ask say this:
"I need to go over the X-rays. I need to do some measurements. I will give you all the options at your consultation visit".

This also shows that you have a system you follow, a strict protocol. You are very thorough in what you do. You don't want to talk about things just like that now.

"I will set aside half an hour or one hour of my time just to meet with you and do just that. I will concentrate on you in that consultation".

Not even a clue of what he needs or what he will expect. But if you are very busy then schedule for the patient before or after your office hours or during lunch.

You take half an hour before or half an hour after the office hours or during lunch just to sit down with the patient and go through this treatment presentation.

Using the Hygiene Appointment

Look at every patient as if he was new.
The hygienist has to go through the file before he or she sees the patient,
-   what has been diagnosed and
-   what has not been done yet.

So there are still some things that have to be done. Then he or she should write that down before he or she meets the patient. Usually at the beginning of the day she should go over the hygiene patients of that day.

Why would she do that? During the hygiene appointment, she re-addresses what has not been done yet. It is important not to contradict the anterior diagnosis. If it has got worse than explain that, "remember last time we told you about this issue? Now it's worse. Now it's very urgent to be addressed ". But only if it really is true, of course.

If it's not true, you still say, "remember what we said last time about this issue? Well, the issue is still there, and it's likely to be worse with time".

And the hygienist can say: "Listen, if you were a new patient, this is what we would tell you to do". All these diagnosed issues that have not yet been done.

If she finds a new issue, she can address that and write it down also, because as soon as the doctor comes in, he will read exactly that piece of paper where he sees the diagnosed things that have not been done yet, and maybe the new issues that she sees, then he makes the exam and addresses all these issues, and it's constant, the patient has been repeated the same things again.

The doctor should be on the same page with the hygienist. That's why you write down this sheet of paper for every patient. And as soon as he comes into the room, he takes that sheet of paper and he is informed about what he should address to the patient.

He should repeat exactly the same things. Consistency is very important.

Time

How much time do you need? It depends on whether it is a small or large treatment presentation. Small presentations need less time, 10 to 15 minutes, large treatment presentations half an hour, or even one hour.

But it depends also on how the attitude of the patient is, is it a fearful patient, then you need more time to explain things and to make him see things like you see them.

You need more time or less time depending on the size of the treatment and the fearfulness of the patient.

During

Then, during the presentation, avoid technicisms, avoid technical terms.

Take the pressure out of yourself. Don't you want them desperately to say yes. If you want them to say yes, you are too stiff. Expect patients to say no or yes. But assume they will say yes. Don't have to be fixed on the idea, that they have to say yes. Assume they will say yes but if they say no, it's okay.

If you fear the "no" you are psychologically in your own way.

Fees

The doctor has to discuss the fees. You will hear, doctors should never discuss fees, doctors should discuss fees.

You should at least give an idea because you are the authority, your fees are set by you. It sounds much more logical and much more acceptable when you, as the authority present the fees, than presented by the front desk manager.

If you say, it's only 500 Euros then it sounds much better for them. This gives credibility to what you say, and to what you have planned. After that, you just say: how would you like to pay for it? Or: how would you normally take care of this?

And you inform that the front desk will explain the different payment option.

Emotions

Dentistry is very emotional. Health, the appearance of the teeth. People smile. That's it's very emotional.

Using needles and drills, scary things, inside of the mouth. Dentistry is very emotional in good things because beautiful smiles enhance your self-esteem, they make you more beautiful, let you have a much better social life. But there are also scary things, negative things involved. So, in both extremes, dentistry is very emotional, and people buy based on emotions and justify with logic.

So, the way they are going to feel, the way people will look at their new smile. These emotions that come up, you have to address these emotions. Let them see the way it's going to make them healthier.

But when they have to pay for it, they need logic to justify the emotions they had when they decided to make the treatment. You need to help them so that it makes logical sense to buy:
- potential consequences. If they see, that if they don't make the treatment something unfavorable is going to happen, then this is a good argument.
- Quality and guarantees,
- your qualifications, your background, your training the training of the staff.

All these things help him or her to justify with logic, the emotional decision of moving forward with your treatment.

Raise the Dental IQ

If patients knew the same about dentistry as a dentist, would case acceptance go up? Of course! If they would know the same thing about dentistry they would accept the treatment option immediately.

Educate them every time you can and use analogies. What's an analogy? Let me explain to you: instead of saying

Occlusion or explain occlusal issues to the patient, you can say, imagine you have a car with four worn-out tires and you replace only three of them. These three will wear out faster than they would have, if you had replaced all four of the tires.

He understands that. If he asks, can you make only the upper teeth? No. Why? Because of this example described as "occlusion".

Filling versus crown. The patient needs a crown, but why not a filling? How do you explain the different things?

Filling in your case would be like using spackle. In some cases it's okay to make a filling. In your case, it would be like using spackle when you in reality need a piece of drywall.

And in your case, a crown would be the solution.

Prophy versus scaling and root planing, which is not the same, of course not, you know it but the patient doesn't know it. Cleaning is like washing your car. Scaling and root planing is like doing bodywork to your car. If your car needs bodywork, and you just take him to the car wash, this is not going to fix the problem.

They understand the examples better if you use analogies. For more analogies, I can recommend a book that is called "Dental Analogies" and it is written by Dr. Waters and Dr. Powell.

Show

During the case presentation, you can show things. And use aids to make the patient understand:

- intraoral cameras
- or you take your mobile phone camera, if you don't have an intraoral camera, you take a mobile phone camera with a LED light ring that clips to the phone, and some intraoral mirrors to make good pictures out of the areas that you want to show. And use a lip retractor. That's all you need.
- Models.
- X-rays,
- Software like DDS GP™ or something like that,
- or short videos on YouTube about the procedures, very short videos, one-minute-videos, half a minute videos, at the most two minutes videos about the procedures so that they see what is going to happen, and then you concentrate on the "whys" of the patient and what happens if we don't do anything about the situation.

Likely

Use the word likely. Make the patients see this:
The condition you have now will *likely* worsen.

You cannot promise that it will get worse. Imagine you said your tooth will get worse and then you will get a root canal and so on. And five years pass and nothing happened to that tooth. What does he think? You're not a good dentist. Of course, you are a good dentist. Of course, what you said will happen, but you cannot say when.

So, and if it did not happen in the next five years, he says: The dentist was not correct in what he said.

Now, in order to make him see what will be going to happen, you don't say "this will happen". You say "this will *likely* happen", "this will *likely* worsen". That's much better.

Open up the person to your proposal

Remember, that you open the mind of people using "just imagine"? Another sentence is:

"How open-minded would you be... to let me show you how..."
-   we fix your teeth,
-   or how we can make your smile really beautiful.

How open-minded would you be? People like to see themselves as open-minded. Nobody admits he is closed-minded.

They immediately would agree. Yeah, I'm open-minded. At that moment, you really opened their mind.

Nobody admits he would be closed-minded. And then you expose your treatment option. And they listen more carefully.

Positive Energy

Be positive, have positive energy during the case presentation, Be happy. Manage your emotions. You transmit it through your tone and body language.

Refocus if you are unhappy, refocus, show the patient, that you are happy. Leave the patient on a happy positive attitude. That's very important to get the "yes".

Help him to lift his mood. He will like you, likability is one of the persuasion principles. Everybody likes to be around mood-lifters.

Avoid yes/no questions

We don't get any information out of that. Instead, ask,

"What do you think will happen if you don't do anything about it?" Or

"Which of the three options do you feel will work best for you?"

Then you get more information about what he needs, what he thinks, what he is concerned about.

First 7 seconds

The first seven seconds are the most important ones. They determine your success.

People judge you about whether or not they
- trust you,
- you are a good guy or a good gal (you're likable),
- you are competent in what you do.

In just about seven seconds. They do that. What can we do to influence their opinion in those seven seconds?
- Nonverbal communication,
- body language,
- eye contact,
- the handshake,
- smile bigger than you think is okay,
- 60 centimeters of space between you and the patient. Don't be a close talker. Nobody likes close talkers. Get away a little bit, in a comfortable distance, don't invade the privacy of 60 centimeters of space. Don't come too near.
- Be present. Be present in your mind the whole time. Show: I'm here to help you.

THE OBJECTIONS

22
YOUR FIRST NO

In this chapter, we will talk about what to do when you get your first "no". We will learn how to change the game and how to use deflection and looping.

Although deflection and looping will come later on in the book again, you will get familiar with these terms.

At first, it's just about when an objection comes up or when a "no" is said to you how you react. First of all, don't panic. You have to change the game.

You get your first no, so what? You should expect that situation. The patient is afraid to buy, that is normal. It's normal to get an objection. An objection in the form of "no" and an objection in the form of "I have to think about it". You should expect that. Act as if you expected it as natural.

Just move forward and be prepared. That is why you have to know how to handle objections and how to close.

This is part of the sales process. How to ask questions is part of the presentation process and patient communication.

When is the worst time to think about what you are going to say? It's when you actually are saying it.

So here comes a "no" and then you have to think, oh, how can I react to that? And the words don't come. You get afraid of the situation, the patient notices that. You make an unprofessional impression. Not good.

The time when you actually are saying it is the worst time to think about what you are going to say. You have to be prepared.

That means you have to have a toolkit of possibilities that you can open, get something out, and put it as a response. Equip yourself with tools and this book is to give you the tools in objection techniques and closing. Learn the objection handling options.

You also have to change your mind, your inner state. You have to be in a positive mind. You have to expect the "no", but also expect that in the end, he will say "yes". Be positive about that.

Be positive about your treatment, about your skills, and your team and your patient service. If you are positive about all this, there is no way he will say "no", in the end.

There is a way to say no at the beginning, in the middle, but not at the end. In the end, he will do it with you, you have to have that confidence. And this confidence, this certainty, (remember, you sell certainty) this certainty is contagious.

Not always, but surely most of the time, the patient says then, let's move forward. You have to change your mind and change your words.

If the patient comes up with a problem, then instead of problems you say: challenge. Because problems are obstacles, and are disempowering and this overwhelms you. It overwhelms the patient if you both see it as a problem.

But if you see it as a challenge it changes the view. Usually to challenges, one raises up. You overcome challenges. It's like a sport.

There are no problems. There are challenges. That is very important. You have to change the game, your attitude, the attitude is everything.

Instead of thinking they will not buy, you have to think they will buy is the greatest thing on Earth, that is why they will buy.

You start with that attitude. Now you are prepared. You expect it, you act as if you expected it. If it would be the most normal thing to do, that everybody says no at that moment.

You are confident and you give the patient that confidence.

You also have to change your mood. Your mind and your mood.

You can be the best closer on Earth. But if you are in a state of uncertainty, if your mood is uncertain, (I don't know today is not a good day. Everything is wrong. I woke up and I stood up with a left leg). That is not good. If you are in that mood, sure, you are not able even to close the door.

It's the same thing if you are a parent. You can be the best parent in the world, but if you are in a state of impatience at that moment, you will not be able (in that moment) to parent or to make good parenting. Everybody understands that.

The same applies to selling. You have to have a good mood at that moment. And if you don't have it, change it, manage it.

Because the patient is now in the chair and you can sell the treatment now, not later now. So be conscious about your state and manage it.

Deflection

The patient makes an objection and you want to put the patient's concerns aside without saying it. That means, you do not make the patient aware of the fact, that you put his objection aside. You don't say, "Well, okay, let's put that aside. But let me explain to you this is this".

That would be rude and insulting for the patient. Deflection is a method to do exactly that. But without saying it. How do you do it? You put the patient's concerns aside and then you go back in a conversation and get him to love your solution. We call that also looping. You go back in a conversation and try another way to explain to him the benefits, because obviously, the way you did it, until now, is not convincing him. How do you know it is not convincing him? He is showing an objection to you.

You have to go back. And once you are back, you can try it again. But to go back first you have to handle his objection.

In the deflection method, you tell the patient that you notice and register his objection. You say,

"I hear or I see what you are saying".

You don't say I understand. This would give him the whole benefit. You say, I hear, I see.
Once you have done that, you go and say,

"but let me ask you a question".

So,

"I hear what you say, but let me ask you a question.
- Does the idea make sense to you?
- Do you love the idea?
- Do you see the idea the same way I see the idea?".

Something like that. That is deflection. This is one of the easiest techniques.

Looping

Looping is to not directly ask why the patient is refusing. If a concern comes up, you have to deal with that concern or that objection. And after that you need to re-explain to the patient why you are the best, why your team is the best and why this treatment is the best for him. Resell your treatment.

Fire the next gun, and at this moment, I have to explain to you a basic idea in the selling process. One basic idea is, that you do not fire all your guns in your presentation. You leave some guns (or also referred to as gunpowder) unfired for the objections later. If you fire all your guns in the presentation and then he comes up with an objection, and you've got nothing else to say anymore because you already fired all the guns, while you were presenting your treatment options, it would not be a good situation.

With guns or gunpowder, we determine the arguments in favor of our offer. The benefits for the patient. Then, when an objection comes up, you deal with the objection. You need to have the instruments of the objection handling chapter. And after that, you loop, you go back and then you fire the next gun.
Example:

"I hear what you are saying.
- And let me say this in another way.
- And let me say this, the real beauty of this treatment is…"
(and then you fire your next gun).

You talk about your next gun.

Usually your guns have to fire on the pain points of the patient. The patient told you what he is running away from, what he doesn't like, and of course "the real beauty" of the treatment is exactly the ability to fix these issues. Then later, you can explain why and how. But first you build up the value again.

If you didn't have enough information, then it did not make sense to move from the questions part into the presentation part.....this mistake provokes objections.

By all means, gather as much information as you can, select your guns and then start the presentation without firing them all, as you will need some of them (probably) for the closing process.

23
A SIMPLE IDEA ON HOW TO
HANDLE OBJECTIONS

In this chapter, we will talk about a simple idea on how to handle objections. It is based on the simple three F idea to follow. You just have to follow these three steps, that are based on three F's. And you can do that every time a patient comes up with any objection. It is very simple.

When a patient comes up with an objection, this is a resistance he is applying. The patient builds up resistance against your offer, your treatment plan, your suggestion.

He is giving you all kinds of objections, doesn't matter what kind of objection, it is an objection.

You need to redirect this energy to get to the close. With this three F method. And here is how it works:

The first F is feel.

Step one, you have to show empathy. But not just fake empathy, but real empathy. You have to understand this objection.

Do not push against the objection. Do not fight it. Don't argue. Instead, try to say this:

"You know what? I understand how you feel". Or "I can see where you are coming from. I understand". You don't have to necessarily use the word feel. Or just "I understand, Yes". Something like that. You have to show real empathy.

The second F is felt.

Step two, let the patient see he is not alone.
"Other patients felt the same way". Or "I felt the same way".
A lot of people have felt the same way, have thought the same way, or had the same problem.

The third F is found.

Step three, show them the solution. "Here is what they found".
These are the people, that had the same feeling, the same problem, the same objection. And this (you show them your treatment solution) is their conclusion.

So: "Dear patient. I understand how you feel, other patients felt the same way. And they found that it was so worth doing this treatment, that they thought they should have done it years before."

This is the three steps way to handle objections. Of course, you don't have to do it like a robot. You have to do it in a natural way. If you train it enough, it comes easily.

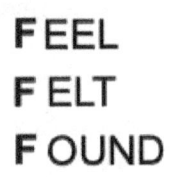

24

MOST COMMON OBJECTIONS
AND HOW TO HANDLE THEM

In this chapter, we will talk about the most common objections and how to handle them. You will learn the basic ideas of objection handling, how to be equipped with tools for any objection, and how to handle the objections in a professional way.

In any possible objection, what you have to do is not to panic, don't worry, don't panic, expect it.

Every patient has a fear of buying, fear of making the wrong decision. Fear of being laughed at because he made a decision that was not okay. So, it is normal, that patients don't want to buy right away.

Objections are just unanswered questions. You have to look at objections as an unanswered question, so you just need to answer them.

In reality, it is not as easy as that. But that is the basic idea. The basic idea is that an objection is an answered question. So it is not something that is a rejection.

Patients are indecisive, a lot of times. You just have to help them through the process to make the correct decision.

That is called objection handling and selling. Whenever they come up with an objection, like,

- I have to talk with somebody,
- I have to think it over.
- The price is too high.
- The treatment is too long, too short.

Whatever objection, then you should behave as if you expected them to say exactly this, although you might have expected something else. The moment he says "the price is too high". And you think that the price is really good, you should behave as if you had expected him to say exactly that.

The basic idea is, you should be convinced that you are the right person to do the treatment and that the treatment is the right thing for this patient, and that your team is the correct team to do altogether that treatment, you and your team.

There are three things the patient has to be convinced of:

- you,
- your treatment and
- your team

You also have to be convinced that you, your team and the treatment are the best things that are going to happen to this patient so that you can help him to make the best decision for him.

Let me think about it

If he says: Let me think about it, in reality, he is saying this: This is a translation of "Let me think about it".
- I don't have the money.
- I don't see the value.
- I don't see the urgency of why I need to buy it right now or why I need to do the treatment right now. I don't see that urgency.
- Based on what you have told me, I don't think it is a good idea for me.

Somehow, summarizing that it means "I don't trust you enough yet". You can change that. There is your opportunity to change it. So, thank God, he is giving you an objection. Now you have the opportunity to change that, to make the trust deeper, bigger, more profound in you, in the treatment, and your team.

How do you do that?

One option is, you can **anticipate** that. If you think, this patient might be a patient that will come up with that sentence, you anticipate or **pre-frame** that.

You say at the beginning of the conversation:

"The purpose of this visit, dear patient, is to see if it is good to do the treatment together, you and us. By the end, you have three things you can say to me:

The first thing is yes, we move forward and that is okay.

The second thing is no. And that is perfectly fine for me. I want you to know if you say no, that is perfectly fine. (Of course, you will take that no. And handle that objection. You will ask him why he says no, and find out his reasons, and then cater to these reasons).

And the third thing you could also say, but I don't want you to say, is: I want to think about it.

So, in my experience, dear patient, what people mean with I want to think about it is No. So, either yes or no at the end of this conversation or the end of this appointment, okay?"

He has to agree on that.

And then you make your presentation, you make your questions, your presentation, and you handle some objections he might come up with, and then you say:

"So, let's move forward (your close). You told me you would tell me if Yes or No. Not Let me think about it."

If he says no, then you can say
"well, it is the money, isn't it?"

Yes. And then you can look for financing options or breaking down the payments, make it easier for him, to get what is good for him: the treatment.

When they say let me think about it in reality they want to say "no". That means you have not given them enough value. Don't confuse price with value. Price is the thing that you made up. You gave the treatment a certain price. You might think now: "I did not give that price. It's the price in my community". Not well done!

If it is the usual price in town or the community, who is dictating your price? The other dentists! *You* should put the price on your treatments, not the other dentists. Nevertheless, somebody came up with that price. And the price is something that can match the value or is over the value or under the value.

The value is individual. For each patient, it's different.

So, if a patient has high urgency and high need, his pain points are so strong, that he wants to go away from that situation and this treatment helps to solve that situation and get him away from that situation, then, the treatment is highly valued by the patient, very high valued.

But obviously, if they say "let me think about it" in reality they want to say no, you have not given them enough value in your treatment. They don't see the value in your treatment for them.

This is why it's so important to ask the questions and to find out their needs, their pain points, urgency, and if they are qualified to pay. You have not qualified them properly, you have to find their needs. And then let them see that exactly these needs are solved with the treatment.

So, <u>the second option</u> is to go back and **loop**. Go back, find his needs, build your value on that. And try to close again after that.

<u>Your price is too high</u>

If they come up with "your price is too high", you have two options.

First, **put the responsibility back** on the patient. How do you do that?
You say: "I agree with you; our price is exactly 200 Euros higher than our next competitor."
And you continue: "Why do you think hundreds of patients have made the treatment with us and not in another clinic?"

Now you put the ball on his roof, he has to answer. Not only that. Now he has to find *your* response to that remark, he has to find out by himself, why the price is not really too high. He is helping you with that.
Maybe he sees value in other things that you did not even think of.

Option number two is to **find out what you miss**. You have to ask yourself: What did I miss? What didn't the patient tell me about how he thinks?
Then you go in to say:

"What makes you say that?"

Maybe like this you find out to whom you are compared. Maybe you are compared to a Dental Chain: "I found Vitaldent™ or XYZ-dent is way lower in the price.

Then you have to start to give value to your service and quality. You can highlight the

- quality material you are using,
- high-end equipment you are using,
- the quality dental technicians you are using,
- the quality instruments you are using,
- how well trained you are,
- how much time you reserve for every patient,
- how your quality control and processes work,...

And all these things, this XYZ-dent might have or might not have. You need to show to the patient that your value is higher, your service is better, your quality is better.

Give me some information to take-away

If they say give me some info to take away, what they want is run away from you. There is an underlying issue.

You say: "I would be more than happy to give it to you. But what exactly do you need?"
Then they have to think about the real objection.
They say one thing.
You say: "Okay, what else?"
With this method, you squeeze out any objection this patient could possibly have.
He says another thing.
You say: "Okay, what else?" You write down.
"Okay, what else?" over and over.
And then you act like in "I'll get back to you".

I'll get back to you

You say: "Let's bottom line this. What would it take for you and me to go forward with the treatment?"

Or you go back and say to this patient, that wanted some information?

"What if I give you the information now? Would you be able to make a decision to move forward with the treatment today?"

"No, I have to talk with my wife."

Aha. There is another thing, okay.

"What if you talk to your wife now? She will love it. Can we get her in?"

She's not here.

"Can we call her, talk to her on the phone?"

All these things can be done.

"What would it take for you and me to move forward with the treatment?"

-   Is it the term?
-   Is it the price?
-   Is it the money that has to be paid? At that moment?
-   What part of the deal you don't like?

"No, everything is fine". This means he is not convinced. You need to find out. What is his objection?

ANY possible objection

You need to clarify the objection.

You need to find out what's the real objection of this patient, and know what he really means.

How do you keep in control of a conversation? When you ask questions. If they give you an objection it is nothing else than an unanswered question and you respond to a question best with another question.

You gain back control of the situation. You have to gain back control of the situation by making a new question.
One possibility for this new question could be:

"What makes you say that?"

You need to ask them why, so you know the real reason or with whom you are compared to, if it is a price issue.

You are too expensive. What makes you say that?
I need to think it over. What makes you say that?
I need to talk with my wife. What makes you say that?

What do they need to tell you now? The rest of the story. What's really behind the objection. In that answer is a detail for you to be able to find the point, the real point of the objection.
And then you help them to see why your treatment, or you or your team are the better choice. By giving them a solution for exactly the real thing that is behind the objection.

What makes you say that? It's not about telling them directly why you are the better choice. This question also buys you time. They gave you an objection, and you don't know what to answer immediately. You say "What makes you say that?" you gain time.
Listen and think about exactly that objection, and what they are now developing, exposing in front of you explaining to you this objection, then you can work on that, as soon as the objection is opened to you.

You can then cater exactly to this open objection, respond to the unanswered questions this objection had hidden behind it.

Objections can be a conflict situation. Be aware that if he says: "You too expensive." and you say "No, that is not true", it generates a conflict okay.

You have to avoid conflict situations if you want to sell. If you want to be an unsympathetic dentist, then you can go ahead and argue with people, but not if you want to be successful in dentistry.

If you respond with an argument, you will end up losing. Maybe you don't lose the argument but you lose the patient or you lose the sale or you lose a treatment and you lose this patient referring other patients to you. Why would you want that? You stand over these things. Don't get into an argument with a patient.

If there is a conflict situation, there is tension and you can reduce this tension in two different ways or with a combination of both ways.

- Either you agree with the patient the tension is gone, or
- you apologize, or
- you agree and apologize.

But what if I disagree?
Wait, you have to remove the fire first.

"The price is very expensive".
"I agree entirely. When I look into buying things I also look for the best possible value".
Notice something? I did not say "price". He's talking about price. You say value, not price. Value! And that is something he can also agree upon. You switch from price to value.
For him the price is an issue, now you make the value an issue. Not the price anymore. And then you continue:
"I am sorry for not explaining myself correctly".

So here we have both ways. We have agreed to the patient and apologized. And then you start explaining the value, don't explain the price.

The price is the price. You have to explain the value. Why your treatment is so valuable by using the best materials, high-end machines, equipment, techniques. For example, "the technique I learned in my continuing education in Dubai in a course of aesthetic dentistry". Something, that gives you more value.

And then, when the patient starts to see that your treatment has a high value and this value goes over the price, then, all of a sudden, the price is not the issue anymore.

Let me explain it to you in a certain way. When you take a Euro banknote, it has written a number on it. Let's say 10. And I say this is a sheet of paper, and I sell this sheet of paper to a patient, for €20 then what would the patient say? No. Why? Because the value of this sheet of paper is written on it. It's 10. I am asking for 20. But it is worth 10, the value is 10. I am asking for too much money for this sheet of paper.

And if I say, I sell you this sheet of paper for one Euro. He says, Okay. Do you have more of these? I buy all of them for one Euro each. The value of this sheet is written on it (10). And the price I said, the first time (20 dollars) was too expensive.

And the second time I said one Euro, that is cheap for this value.

Good news. The value of our treatments is not written on veneers or on the bleaching itself. It's not written, we can create the value, we can make the patient see that there is a lot of value behind our treatment. The price will always be lower than the value if we manage to transmit enough value the right way.

Then find out if that is the only objection he has, because you don't want to go forth and back and forth and back the whole time with any objections.

"Is that the only thing that bothers you about this treatment?"
No, there is another thing
"What is it?"

We can handle three objections, but four, five, or six... maybe you are speaking to the wrong patient. In this case, you stop there and you say, I probably cannot help you with that problem. Because if he has so many objections on your treatment, maybe you are not the right person, or your team is not the right one or the treatment that you are offering is not the correct one for this patient.

In any possible objection, change your mind about the words they use.

If they say:
"I need to talk to my partner".
You have to hear:
"I need to talk to my partner because it's fantastic".

If they say:
"It's too expensive"
You have to hear:
It's too expensive, but I love it.

If they say:
"I need more time to think"
You have to hear:
"I need more time to think because you gave me more than I can understand right now. And it sounds so good. I don't know what to do next".

That is why they need more time. You don't have to think it's negative, think always it is positive.
This thinking makes your attitude towards this person not a defensive one. But an attitude that is an embracing one, you

embrace the objection, you embrace the person that makes the objection.

Objections are an opportunity for you to tell patients better, what you can do. Thank God, there is an objection.

Because otherwise, maybe he was not completely convinced of everything. If he's not convinced and he doesn't give you an objection. It's not good to sell.

Here are the steps again:

- You have to clarify the objection by making a question.
- Then you agree or apologize, or you agree and apologize.
- Is this objection the only one? You find out if there are more objections, listen to the objection positively. Think it is a reason to buy and not a reason not to buy.
- Tell them what you can do and not what you can't do. If you feel the patient is not yet ready, or he has another objection, then you go back and loop.
- You go back and sell him on you, on your team, and the treatment. If you feel the patient is ready, and he has no objections, then you can move towards the easy next step that you know is right for him.
- You close and there all the closing techniques come into the game.

SPECIAL SITUATIONS

25
WHEN THE PATIENT ASKS

In this chapter, we will talk about how to respond when the patient asks. Learn the most common questions and how to react to them during your presentation.

How much is it?

One of the questions could be, how much is it? It depends on where we are at the presentation, we respond or we react to the question differently.

If we are at the beginning of the presentation, and the patient asks this question, then it means they want to get to the bottom line immediately, and they don't care about features benefits. They don't want to know what you can do for them. They want to know how much it is.

If you tell the price now, you lose control. Imagine you tell the price and he says no, then you go into justification mode. All of a sudden you have to justify why you need to charge that price. Don't do that. Instead of that, the idea is to create value. And then, at the end mention the price. When the value is higher, not at the beginning. At the beginning, you would mention the price and then justify it. That's not the ideal situation. But how can you not respond to that question? Let me explain to you how you handle that.

If you get that question at the beginning of your presentation. Redirect the conversation. Go back to the needs. You say:

"It depends". And then you address the need.

"It depends. What exactly do you need?" or,

- what exactly are you looking for? Or
- what exactly do we need to accomplish here?

If the patient asks <u>at the end of the presentation</u>, how much is it? You had enough time to create the value. You already have qualified him. Imagine you know that he needs it. It's the best for him. He wants it. He can pay for it. You have qualified him through your questions, you have found out that he is okay to move forward.

Then, but only then, you say the price and you say it confidently like this:

"It's only 5000 Euros". Use always the word 'only'. And then ask a question immediately, so that the attention of the patient is redirected from the number of Euros you said to a minor decision problem (start Monday or Wednesday for example).

"It's only 5000 Euros when would you like to start?" or

"It's only 5000 Euros? How would you like to pay for it?"

If it is <u>in the middle of the presentation</u>, you did not have enough time to ask all the questions that you need to ask, to see if the patient sees it the same way as you see the situation. He interrupts your flow. He answered to one of your questions, but then immediately asks the question "How much is it?" before you make the next question. You still have not explained the value well enough. You can now give him a range, it's between 200 Euros and 500 Euros.

And then you ask the next question, the question that you would have asked anyhow. It is between here and here. And I need to know more to tell you exactly the price. Don't say that last sentence that I wrote. But it is a logical continuation of this range. You say a range and after this range, you ask a question. The next question to qualify him, the next question you would have asked anyhow.

Do you have a guarantee?

Another question that the patient can come up with, is. do you have a guarantee? Don't assume what he means with 'guarantee'. Don't take it so literally. Don't justify if you don't have one.

Instead answer with a question. For example,
You say: you need a prophylaxis.
He says: Do you have a guarantee? (guarantee for a prophylaxis?)
You say: We don't.

Don't assume anything. Instead answer with a question. By the way. One ground rule, who is always in control of a conversation? It's always the one who asks questions. He can direct the conversation in different directions through the questions.
"Exactly what kind of guarantee are you looking for?"
Now you are not assuming something, they tell you their concern, "what if my teeth are sensitive afterward?" That's what he meant. Or how long will my mouth stay without tartar?
"It depends" and then you can address these issues.

These are only concerns they don't know how to ask you certain things. So, they come up with the 'guarantee' thing. You can now answer their concerns and say,
"is that what you're looking for?" Or
"are you comfortable with that?"

Or you can say, "suppose we have a guarantee. What would that look like for you?" You are not guessing. They tell you their concern. "So, suppose we have that, what's going to happen next?". Maybe they come up with another concern. So, it was not really the guarantee what bothered them.

You ask what guarantee they are thinking of and you address their concerns. And if it was a guarantee, you address the concerns and then move forward to make the next step which would be to accept the treatment.

Can you give me a discount?

Don't do that. Don't lower your fees. Please don't lower your fees.

The first thought of the patient if you lower your fee by 20%, is "I knew he was overcharging". Now, think of in what light does this leave you? What does he think about you? That you are a professional person? No, more like "you're a dubious second-hand-car-salesman, and you wanted to overcharge me and now because I asked for a discount, you go down to the price that you really should have asked for from the beginning".

I know you want to help the patient maybe. But don't do that. This means, everybody else is being overcharged in his mind. Don't make a discount. You would not appear honest or genuine. And, believe me, definitely for your own branding it's good to appear honest and genuine.

And it's unprofessional. You look like an unprofessional guy. Why didn't you put your prices so high, if you can go down, you showed that you can go down.

Much better is to prove and show that you cannot go down. Say: "If you want the cheapest dentist in town, I'm not your guy. I'm so sorry". And then don't send him out of the office. Just explain the differences in material
- that you are using the highest quality material and

- that you are using the highest quality equipment.
- The facility you are in is very expensive in a very easy to access area in a high-level area of town.
- The constant continuing education you are taking. And all the books you read, for example, this book.
- The dental technician you are using, who is a higher-level than other technicians.
- Your team training.

All these things differentiate your office from other offices and your prices from other prices. Explain them.

What you can do is to maybe offer our 5% paid in full in advance courtesy. I am not a big fan of that, but at least it is not a discount. That is just to help him decide to do it immediately and to get a commitment of this person, he pays all in advance, and then for that, you make a 5% courtesy.

And this is sort of giving him something and not leaving him without anything. But it's not like lowering your prices.

Why is this so expensive?

Another question. A very similar question is: why is this so expensive?

Clearly you haven't built enough value for the patient at that moment. If your value is high, and your price is lower than the perceived value for the patient, then he will never ask, why is this so expensive? Because it's less expensive than the value you are offering.

Maybe you think you build value by explaining the procedure, but maybe for him, it's not valuable, what you are explaining. That is why you have to find out his needs and his wishes. The "why". Why does he want to make the treatment and this makes him see the value in your treatment. If you say, this treatment makes you feel like this, or makes us fix that problem, that problem is exactly the one problem that he was thinking of, then it has a high value. If it fixes many, many other problems that have no value for that patient, (maybe have value for other patients, but not for that patient), then he will not move forward.

It's important to understand these concepts. Because something might be valuable for you, it does not have to be necessarily also valuable for the patient.

Ask a patient what is important for him and then create value or let him see that the treatment that you are offering is exactly solving the problem that he wants to be solved.

Price is what you pay.
Value is what you get.
(Warren Buffet)

Remember this always. When you are talking to a patient, you are not talking about the price, you are talking about the value.

What is in for the patient? What does the patient get?

The value! The price is what he pays.

26
THE INDECISIVE PATIENT

In this chapter, we will talk about the indecisive patient. You will learn two different options to handle that situation: the sudden death close and tell them what to do in a smooth way.

Sudden Death Close

The option one is the sudden death close. It's also discussed in the closing strategies chapter. It is a technique you use as an ultimatum.

Imagine you've seen the patient several times. He has come in two or three times for information about certain treatment, smile make-over, periodontal treatment, whatever. And you have seen him several times, but he won't give you an answer yes or no.

What you do is you fill out the entire Informed Consent Agreement with all details except the signature of the patient.
You even put the date of today. And then you put it on the table in front of the patient. And you say:

"Mr. patient, we have discussed this quite a bit now. And I know this is taking up a lot of your time" (*your* time, you think about the patient, that is what you want to transmit).

"It's taking up a lot of my time as well.
And either this is a good idea for you, or it's not.
So, one way or another. Let's make a decision right now.
 What do you say?"

And then you give him the pen to sign the informed consent.
That is how you do the sudden death close. You gently push him towards the close.

<u>Tell them what to do (in a smooth way)</u>

The second option is you tell them what to do. Nobody likes to be told what to do. So be careful.

How do you tell somebody what to do? We want to tell them what to do. But you can't tell them what to do because it would be rude and pushy to tell them what to do.

You need to give them the confidence that other patients like them have acted in a similar way before them. And you want them to feel like it was their idea, and you didn't influence their decision in any way. But, of course, it was your idea. Of course you *did* influence them. But you don't want them to feel that.

They have to think they made up their own mind without any pressure from you. It's not true. You use a technique.

You tell them

"what most people would do",

this is a very important sentence.

You say,

"What most people would do in your situation is they would go for... (the in-office whitening and then the upper six front veneers), that is what most people would do".

That's it. That is not: "I recommend you to do", "I tell you what to do", "I push you towards doing this and this".

No, although you do that also, although the message is the same, you deliver it in a different way. You tell them what *most* people would do.

It's not *your* decision. It's the decision of others. So you just tell him what others would do, and he starts to think: "I am most people. The doctor is not going to tell me what to do. I'm going to do my own mind up and I'm going to do exactly that what most people would do. I go for it".

My experience tells me

Some patients might think I'm **not** most people. Don't worry if they say that. You say:

"What is best for your situation? Based on what you told me, my experience tells me that this and this solution is the best for your situation".

Notice something? "my experience tells me" not, "I tell you", it's my experience that tells me this.

Do you get the difference in the presentation of the options for the patient?

Back to "what most people would do". Literally most people will think: "oh, good idea. I do what most people will do".

Does it work with all the patients all the time? Of course not.

But it works with most indecisive patients most of the time for those patients, where it doesn't work, you use the other possibility of "my experience tells me".

27
THE ANGRY PATIENT

In this chapter, we will talk about how to communicate with an angry patient. You will learn to understand the most common causes, why patients get angry, and learn different strategies on how to react to them. I will also explain to you two different separate strategies with different steps. One eight-step strategy and a 10-step strategy and then very common things of how to de-escalate the situation.

6 reasons why patients are dissatisfied

There are six main reasons why patients are dissatisfied.

- Bad experience at the front desk,
- Long wait in the reception area,
- Unattractive practice
- Can't get a timely appointment
- The office doesn't accept their insurance
- The hygienist is a stabber.

Bad experience at the front desk

Visiting a dentist is no fun. So, if the patient is not greeted with a warm "Hello" and a smiling face, he starts doubting whether he chose the right office. A bad start means the sabotage of the rest.

You can be a very good closer and a very good presenter. If the beginning was not good, then everything is much more difficult.

Long wait in the reception area

Time is precious. Waiting 10 minutes or more is not acceptable. It upsets the patient and frustrates him. So, let them know if you are behind schedule. If you know beforehand, you can call the patient before he comes and says, "we are more or less half an hour behind schedule. If you want you can come half an hour later or we can reschedule your appointment". If you are more than 20 minutes behind, let them reschedule if they want to. Show you care about the patient.

Unattractive Office

Do you have an unattractive practice? The look of your office is a reflection of the care you deliver.

How are the toilets? Are they clean? Do they smell well? Is everything in the right place? Are they nicely looking?

I know this has nothing to do with your clinical skills. But patients look at these things and make assumptions that are not logically connected. And they assume your clinical skills are as horrible as your toilets are or as horrible as your clinic looks, like cabinets, reception area, windows, ceiling, lamps, and many more things.

Can't get a timely appointment

The best is to get a new patient in, the first 48 hours after he called. Maximum one week after, they should be sitting in your chair, and emergencies maximum 24 hours later. Otherwise, they might leave the office, they go to another office. They just don't wait.

You don't accept their insurance

If you accept insurance, then evaluate the percent of your patients that have that insurance before you drop that insurance. If you never had any, then you can tell the patient always.

"We don't work with X insurance, but many of our patients have exactly this insurance and come in because they value the high quality and the good service that we give".

This is the standard sentence we say to all the calls, that ask for insurance. We convert still nearly 60% of these people to patients.

Your hygienist is a stabber

Change her. Survey your patient experience ask them always if everything went well. You can use surveymonkey.com for that. Does she turn the gum into a pin-cushion? Well, that's not fun.

It reinforces old perceptions and old concepts of dentistry and you want to be a modern dentist or a modern clinic. His or her hands are a prolongation of your (the doctor's) hands.

If she is a stabber, patients assume you are a butcher. So, change your hygienist.

If a patient is angry

So, if a patient is angry, you should first apologize. Mistakes happen to all of us. That's human life and thoughtless comments can escalate the situation.

So, first you apologize. You might think: "But it's not my fault". Nevertheless, you apologize. Defensiveness and blame intensify that the patient is angry.

Learn to see each problem as an opportunity for improvement.

Eight steps to deal with difficult patient situations.

Step one: Listen

Don't downplay the seriousness of the patient's complaint. "You only waited for 10 minutes. Oh, that's nothing". No, don't do that. You listen. You pay attention or the front desk listens and pays attention.

Let them tell you their side of the story. No interruptions. If you interrupt an angry patient, he gets angrier.

Sometimes all they need is to be heard.

Step two: Empathy

Show empathy. Let them know you understand the problem. And you are concerned about their feelings. This is important for the patient to have the impression, that he has been understood by you.

Step three: Be okay

Patients need to hear that you are on their side, and that you are willing to whatever it takes to solve the problem.

That does not mean you agree on the fact, that the office or you have caused the problem.

You just understand the problem, and you signal to the patient that you want to solve the problem. It does not mean you admit that you provoked the problem.

Step four: No confrontation

Don't go on defensive mode. With confrontation, you lose the patient. Instead, you should use endorsement softeners and say:
-   I appreciate that.
-   I see / I hear.
-   Thank you for sharing.
    What else do I need to know about that?
-   I know how you feel, others have felt that way, too, and they found... this what we can do and they had a really good result.

Step five: Take action

Once you have heard the story, take control. You make the plan, you say where we are going to.
And you take action to start to resolve the problem.

Step six: Ask

Ask the patient what he wants. Sometimes his solution is both fair and simple. If you don't ask you don't know what the patient really wants.
-   I am committed to making this work.
-   How can I support you?
-   Would that work for you?
-   I believe this and that, and I could be wrong.

Step seven: Plan

Establish a plan of action and sell it to the patient so that he is okay with that plan. Explain how the plan will solve the problem.

Step eight: Follow up

Make sure the plan is carried out. Make sure the results are acceptable for the patient. Follow up with the team, with the patient and/or with somebody who did solve his problem.

The second approach is a 10 ways approach

It is very similar to the first approach, but it has some different issues.

Step one: Listen

Listen with concern and empathy. Let them tell you their side of the story, no interruptions. Sometimes all they need is to be heard.

Step two: Isolate the patient

Isolate him if possible, so that other patients won't overhear what he says and describes.

Step three: Stay calm

Don't argue with the patient.

Step four: Be aware of the patient's self-esteem.

They really get bigger and bigger. Show a personal interest in the problem. Try to use the patient's name frequently. People like to hear their name, that shows also empathy.

Step five: Attention

Give the patient your undivided attention. Concentrate on the problem. Not on placing blame, or searching who is to be blamed. Do not insult the patient.

Step six: Take notes.

Writing down the key facts saves time if somebody else has to be involved. If somebody else in the office should solve the problem of the patient, then it helps to have some notes, and also, the patient tends to slow down when they see somebody typing, or writing down the issue. They understand you pay attention and you take it seriously.

Step seven: Tell

Tell the patient what can best be done. Offer choices, but don't promise the impossible.

Step eight: Set a time

Set an appropriate time for the completion of corrective actions. Be specific, but do not underestimate the amount of time it will take to resolve the problem.

Step nine: Monitor

Monitor the progress of the corrective action.

Step ten: Follow up

Even if the complaint was resolved by somebody else, you follow up. That shows that you are personally interested. Contact the patient to ensure that the problem was resolved to his full satisfaction.

Words to be used with Arrogant Patients

To handle better difficult situations, different types of patients need to hear different types of words. With arrogant patients use words like:
- We appreciate your opinion a lot.
- Can we do something *special* for you?
- You certainly know about the subject, *and* I have special information.
- We find out where the mistake was.
- This is certainly very important.
- Your opinion or critics is very important for us.
- You are very important to us.
- We try the best for you.
- What do you think about this?
- I share your opinion.
- Your treatment is very important.

All these things slow down or de-escalate the arrogant patient.

Words to be used with Aggressive Patients

An aggressive patient is slowed down with other words:
- You are obviously very angry.
- This has made you for sure very angry.
- I can imagine how angry you are. (But don't just say it, show with your body language and with your tonality that you can imagine).
- Can we speak calmly about it?
- We'll check exactly where the mistake has been made.
- Can you describe exactly what makes you so angry?
- Probably I would be angry, too in this situation.
- Good that you have told us about it.
- We take your disappointment very seriously, please tell me what makes you so angry.

De-escalation Strategies

De-escalation strategies help to de-escalate the situation and to redirect the conversation. They help to make the patient less angry and to solve the problem. Several strategies can be used.

Acknowledging without Encouraging

Let them know you understand.
Empathy statement combined with refocusing away from emotions, back to the problem. You say: I understand, and then you show empathy.

I understand that you are very angry
I understand the problem
I understand that you have to be very angry right now

and then you refocus away from these emotions towards the problem.

What is exactly the problem and how can we solve it now?

Allowing Venting

You just allow the patient to set off the steam uninterrupted. They will eventually calm down. Except for obsessors, they will get angrier and angrier. They will enter into a vicious cycle of angriness.

If you see the patient is allowed to vent and calms down, good. If you see the patient is allowed to vent and gets angrier and angrier, then he needs an empathy statement and refocusing.

Allowing venting does not work for everybody.

Apologize

That does not necessarily mean you are admitting culpability. You apologize and then refocus and solve the problem.

I am so sorry that you feel like this. (You are not sorry that you made a mistake).

You apologize anyhow and then, followed by an assurance of effort, or of result. You let them know you will do your best to meet his or her needs.
If you assure results, give a guarantee for the result.

Audience Removal

You take the patient away from the audience. It's not easy to make, but some angry patients will play to the audience. They get angry again, and they see people looking, so they get more and more and shout more so that everybody is involved in the waiting room.

You don't want that to happen. Take them to an office space. You say: "Mr. patient, I'm sure you'd prefer your privacy is protected. Let's go to the office. We can continue there".

You make clear, it is something you do for *them* and not for any other reason.

Distraction

There are different ways to distract the patient. You shift the attention of the patient away from the anger and away from expressing the anger to you.

This strategy is designed to break the anger-cycle. You direct their attention to a physical object with words and gestures, for example. And then they have to break eye contact with you.

"If you see here in the screen...", and then you show the patient the screen, then the patient instead of looking to you, looks at the screen that stops and breaks the cycle of anger.

Instead of the screen, any physical object relevant to the subject will do. A brochure, a sign, a paper, something written in a paper or brochure.

"If you can see here the informed consent..."
'If you can see here', so the patient focuses there, and then you can go on with the solution.

Not taking the Bait

If he insults you, don't respond with insults.
If he is angry, don't respond with anger. Don't take the bait. Be empathetic.

Refocus

"I can see you're angry because of XYZ.
Let's go back to what we can do to help you"

Refocus on helping, not on the anger, not on the cause, but to how we can help the patient. Then you say:

"I can suggest a few things".

And then you go ahead explaining your solution.

Use of Timing

When you use the other strategies, sometimes angry patients are not able to think logically yet. If they are not ready, no technique will work.

First, they need acknowledgment and empathy. Only if he is less angry you have to move forward with other de-escalation strategies.

How do you know? It is too early, if he is ignoring your attempts, and you have to repeat yourself because he is not hearing you. Then it would be too early.

Then you will have to acknowledge, apologize, and refocus. That's what they need to hear.

OTHER BOOKS FROM THE AUTHOR

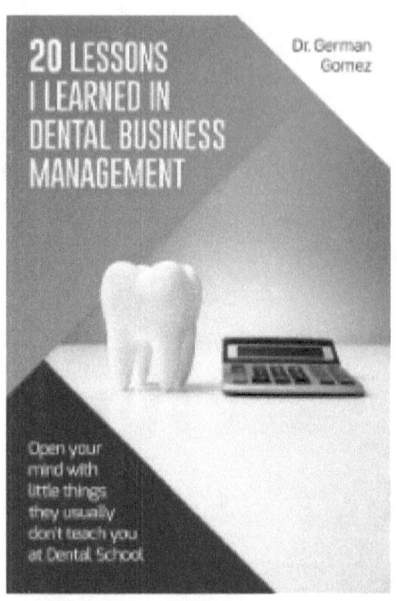

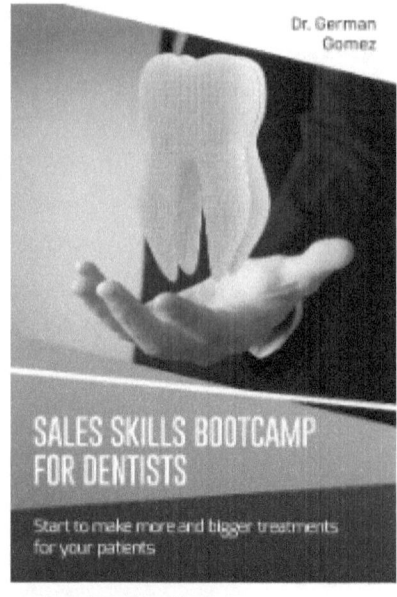

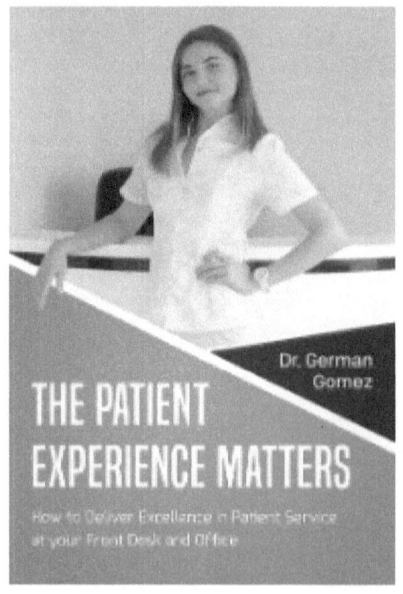

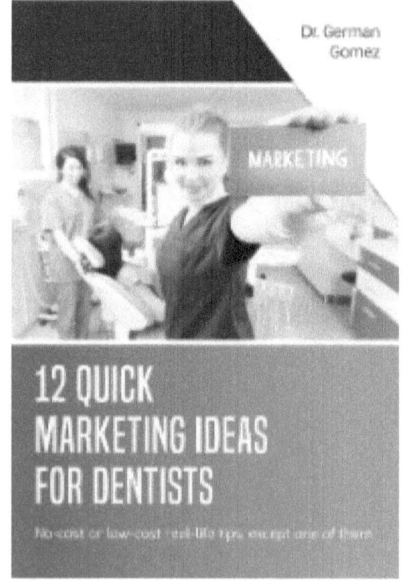

www.ingramcontent.com/pod-product-compliance
Lightning Source LLC
Chambersburg PA
CBHW030624220526
45463CB00004B/1402